WALK
YOURSELF
FIT

Happy Fitwalking!

David A. Rives

WALK
YOURSELF
FIT

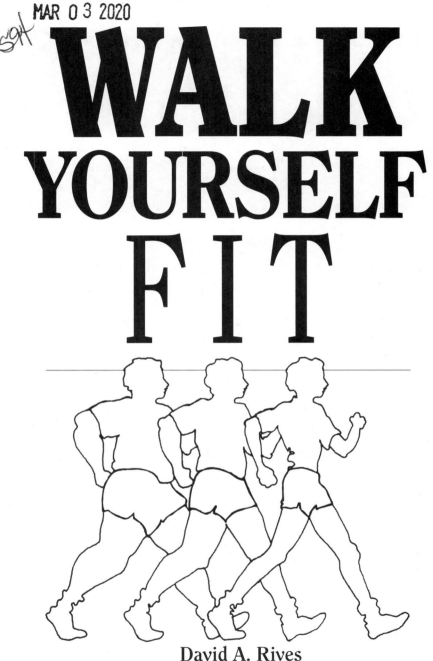

David A. Rives
Author of *Dying for a Smoke*
Illustrations by David Levi

First Edition (revised), © 2019 by Moon River Publishing

"Walk Yourself Fit;" "Fitwalk;" "Fitwalker;" "Fitwalking;" are all trademarks of

Moon River Publishing
812 Natchez Avenue
Liberty, MO 64068
(800) 522-7735
e-mail: davidrives@hotmail.com

10 9 8 7 6 5 4 3 2 1

978-1-878143-02-0

If nothing changes,
Nothing changes.

Zen bumper sticker

This above all: To thine own self be true.

Hamlet

Preface

This book was written to help otherwise-healthy people get a little fitter and lose a little bodysize (formerly known as "weight"), and to do so by walking, rather than by another in the seemingly-endless succession of "diets" most of us have been on for the last hundred years or so, with no long-term benefit that I can see!

As a result, we had no problem telling such people:

"We don't care what you eat. As long as you walk it all off, you **will get fit** and **may lose bodysize.**"

Unfortunately, in a world of 7 billion people, not everyone will be "otherwise healthy." Rather, we will have people with special health needs in our midst—diabetics, heart patients, etc.—who **can't** eat "everything under the Sun," even if their **neighbors** can.

For you people, all we can say is: when you come across parts of the book that tell you you can eat whatever you want, whenever you want it, please understand that those parts do not apply to you.

Instead, we would ask you to simply ignore those parts and eat only what and when your health professional **tells** you to eat.

Thanks.

Table of Contents

1

All Aboard!

You're about to set off on a remarkable journey; a "walking tour" of a wonderful new world, where you will:

• Get fit forever—and lose some bodysize—without having to put out a zillion dollars for gym memberships, skiing trips, etc.
• Take the part of your mind that makes you eat and turn it into your **best friend** for a change, instead of your **worst enemy**, the way all "diets" do!
• Feel **better** and **better** as you get fitter and trimmer.
• Finally start enjoying all the wonderful things fit, trim people enjoy, **just because they're fit and trim**!

Just Fitwalk for one enjoyable hour a day and you'll give yourself a body you can be even prouder of, a body you'll want to look at, put clothes on, take out in public, share with others even **more** than you do now.

The streets and running tracks of America are filling up with Fitwalkers (people walking themselves fit and trim)—all knowing the joy of eating all the good food they want, then burning off any extra calories.

We invite you to join us on those streets, that track, to begin a life you've only dreamed of; a life that is finally yours for the taking; a life of Fitwalking!

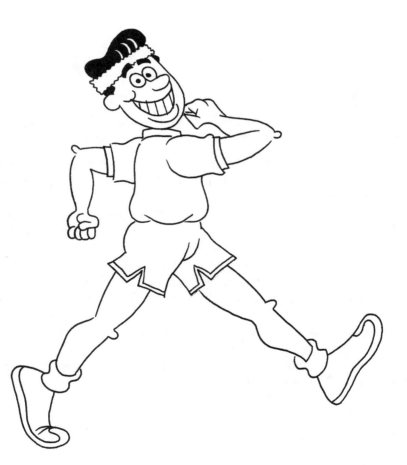

2

Before you Start

You're about to walk yourself fit. Which means you're going to have to change your lifestyle a teensy, tiny bit— take a more active role in shaping your own future.

Because of that, and because the lawyers inform me this world has gotten kind of sue-happy lately, there's one thing I've got to tell you:

Like any program where you have to move a tad faster than a glacier, you could be looking at a possible health risk here.

So, before you do anything, you really should tell your family doctor what you're about to do—get his "seal of approval."

And now that we've covered our rear ends with the standard "see-your-doctor" routine, you want to know what we **really** think about it?

We hate it!

Why?

Oh, not because it isn't necessary; it is!

It's just that Fitwalking is such a mild exercise that very few of you will wind up on the wrong side of an oxygen tent because of it.

So the next time it comes down to a choice between, say, "cookies" and "walking," you might want to see what "walking" can do for you—doctor or no doctor—since there can't be all that many surprises left for you in that cookie jar of yours!

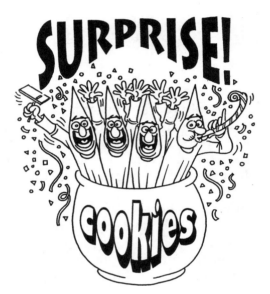

It's amazing: someone like Sara Lee never has to tell you to "see a doctor" before you eat any of **her** stuff. And yet, her stuff makes people plus-sized, and plus-sized people seem to leave us a whole lot sooner than normal-sized people do, if I've been reading those insurance charts right. And yet, she gets **awards** for her stuff, while "exercise pushers" have to tiptoe past courtrooms!

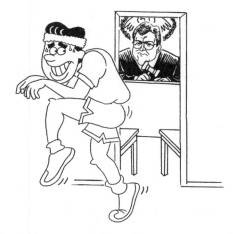

I guess old Sara figures we're all smart enough to know that we should "take" her products in teensy, tiny "doses," and that if we abuse those products, that's **our** problem, not hers. Which, of course, is the same thing you hear from liquor companies, and tobacco companies, and wine companies, and beer companies, and anyone else selling something so drop-dead addictive!

And, since those billionaires all seem to get away with it, I guess they're right: it **is** our fault! Wow: shame on **us**!

Now me, all I'm "selling" is "health." So I've got to warn you that if you do what you were given a body to do—move around—so you can get that body functioning even better than it is now, you might be the one-in-a-million who shouldn't have. And the only way we're going to know that is if you let your doctor check you out.

So do it.

But while you're waiting for him to check **you** out, you might want to take a minute or three and check **us** out as well; you know: put one foot in front of the other for a block or two.

Why?

Because then, if "Doc" says you're **not** that one-in-a-million, you'll already be that many miles closer to a Beautiful New You!

3

"Vive la Difference!"

Before you start, we've got to tell you one thing:
"What's that?"
You can forget about losing weight with Fitwalking.
"What?!"
That's right.
"See ya!"
No, don't leave! Hear us out!
"Wel-l-l-l....."
That's better.

All we're saying is that Fitwalking isn't a typical weight-loss program—what you would call a "diet." It's an **exercise** program, and exercise programs work differently than "diets:"

Every day, your body has to burn a certain number of calories to keep you alive and kicking. Feed your body **fewer** calories than it'll be burning—the way you do on every "diet"—and the only place the body can go to for the missing calories is the fat it's been storing, every time you've had one-too-many Twinkies!
In other words: Feed your body a pound's-worth of calories when it needs to burn two, and, with any luck, your body will pull a pound of fat out of storage and burn that to make up the shortfall.
So what's different about Fitwalking?

Only everything:

Oh, not the part about fat-burning; that stays the same. It's the **reason** for the fat-burning that changes:

With the "diet," you burned fat to make up for some calories you didn't eat; with Fitwalking, you burn fat to build up leg muscles you've been exercising.

So what?

Well, with the "diet," you had only one thing happening: a pound of fat disappearing, which meant you lost a pound of weight.

With Fitwalking, two things happen: that pound of fat still disappears, but now a pound of new muscle shows up in its place!

"So?"

So at the end of each Fitwalking day, instead of being "one pound 'short,'" like you were on your "diet," you find that you're "**no** pounds 'short'"—but you're still one "pound" **skinnier**!

"Wait a minute: how can that be? How can I be skinnier without losing any weight?"

Easy: because

A pound of muscle takes up a lot less space than a pound of fat.

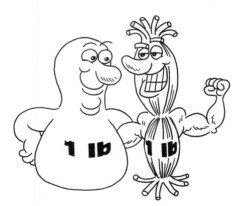

So every time you "trade" a pound of fat for a pound of muscle, like you do with Fitwalking, you lose a lot of **size** without losing any **weight**!

"Oh-h-h."

That's why we tell you to forget about losing weight with Fitwalking, because you probably **won't** lose any—especially when you first get started.

All you'll lose is body **size**—great, gobbing hunks of bodysize—and you'll lose it more easily, more permanently and more naturally than you ever did on any "diet."

This may be hard to take at first—losing size without losing weight—but as you grow more and more gorgeous, you'll learn to live with it.

Every other Fitwalker has!

4

"Let's Take a Walk"

One thing you can't avoid: If you're going to get fit—and lose some bodysize—you're going to have to **control** something: either your "gonzo" eating or your (apparently) less-than-"gonzo" exercising.

Since no one on this planet seems to want to control **anything** anymore, we'd be kind of stupid to pick the one that's the **hardest** to control!

"Which is?"

Well, how do you feel about giving up your omelets and muffins and cookies and candy and rolls and butter and french fries and pizza and—

"STOP IT!"

That's what we thought. Next question: Any problem taking a nice refreshing walk every day?

"None that I can think of."

Fine. And since that "nice refreshing walk" will get you just as fit and trim as giving up all the food in Fargo, why torture yourself?

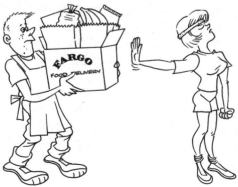

"Hey, you've got **my** vote! When do we start?"

Very soon.

"One question, though:"

Yes?

"Why 'walking?' Why not 'jogging?' Or 'swimming?' Or 'skiing?' Or 'biking?' I mean, all you're talking about is 'exercising yourself fit,' right?"

Right.

"So what difference does it make **which** exercise you choose?"

Makes no difference at all—as long as you choose the **best** one.

"Which is...?"

Well, why are we talking exercise in the first place?

"So we can build a little muscle and lose a little bodysize."

Very good. So what would an exercise have to do to be the "best" exercise?

"I guess: be the one that builds the **most** muscle, and helps us lose the **most** bodysize."

That's right. And not just "per session," but "per year/decade/millennium/etc."

And what would keep biking or swimming or jogging or skiing from being the best exercise?

Well, how much time do you think overweight joggers spend, nursing injuries? Exactly!

See a lot of skiers when there's no snow, do you?

Oh, it was **water** skiing you were referring to? Terrific exercise! All you need is a body of water and a boat and a driver and a line and skis and a lovely Summer's day and—

Swimming? There's that "body of water" again!

Biking? No problem: as long as you have a bike and it's actually working.

You get the picture: an exercise isn't much good if you're not doing it. And if there's a million reasons **not** to do something, chances are awfully good you won't. Which means you won't be building any muscle and won't be losing any bodysize

And what's to stop you from walking? Well, aside from the obvious—blizzards, hurricanes and the like—nothing comes to mind. All you have to do is strap on a decent pair of shoes, dress appropriately and step out your front door (or stay inside and hop on a treadmill).

So, at the end of a year's time, who do you think will have built more muscle and lost more bodysize: the running/ skiing/swimming/biking "hare"—who spends more time on the "shelf" than on the "mark"—or the Fitwalking "tortoise," who just takes a nice brisk walk every day—day after day after day after day...............?

"Silly question!"

So who's done the "best" exercise?

"Let's go 'turtle' on this one."

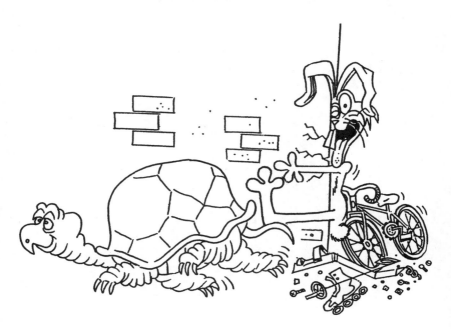

So, if you're using Fitwalking to get a little slimmer—as well as build a little muscle—forget about how good an exercise looks on paper: "**Burn Seven Million Calories an Hour, Cross-country Skiing!**"; the paper's **already** slim!

Just go out and Fitwalk every day and you'll burn more calories—and lose more bodysize—than all the skiers, bikers, joggers, and swimmers **combined**!

Of course, as you walk yourself fit, you'll start to feel so good, so "energized," that you'll be "chafing at the bit" to do some of those other exercises.

So—DO THEM! Do every one of them you think you might enjoy!

Just one thing, though:

Don't do any of them to **get** fit; do them only after you **are** fit. That way, you won't jeopardize your Get-fit Program halfway through by switching from an exercise you can and will do every day—Fitwalking—to an exercise you can't or won't.

Other than that: Exercise away! As you'll soon discover: that's what getting fit is all about!

5

"Fitwalking"

Oh sure: 'walking.' Know all about it. Been doing it all my life!"

Fine. But if you're not as fit and trim as you'd like to be, we'll bet you haven't been walking fast enough or far enough for your walking to be classed as "exercise."

And how fast and how far would that be?

Well, to turn "walking" into "Fitwalking," all you have to do is

WALK AS FAST AS YOU COMFORTABLY CAN FOR AS LONG AS YOU COMFORTABLY CAN!

"That's it?!"

That's it.

"Doesn't sound like much."

Oh, but it is:

1) When you walk as fast as you **comfortably** can (and that speed will change every minute you're walking), you'll always be burning the **most fat calories you can**; go any slower and you won't be burning the "max;" go any faster and you risk burning **yourself** out, long before you had any need to.

13

2) By walking only as **long** as you comfortably can, you'll always be building the most muscle and burning the most fat calories you can **at each session**, without jeopardizing your **next** session by "overdoing" it.

Since you never **lose** any sessions, you wind up building the most muscle and burning the most fat calories you can— per year, decade, millennium, etc.—which is how you get fit and stay fit.

A word of advice, though:

No matter how fast you'll be going at the peak of your walk, always start out slowly and work up to that peak gradually. That way, your muscles won't "burn out" sooner than they should have, leaving calories on your body and not on the road or track where they "belong!"

When you begin your Fitwalking program, your legs may feel sore at the start of each session. Not to worry: that soreness will work its way out as you walk, so don't ever let that temporary soreness keep you on the couch.

In fact, a lot of people tell me they wind up having their **best** Fitwalking sessions on days they've felt their **worst** going in: "tired," "listless," "ache-y," etc. I don't know why this is so; it just is.

And because it is, you should always think twice before passing up a Fitwalk just because you "don't feel like it." If so, you could be cheating yourself out of a fun workout, and, more important, keeping Fitwalking from doing its job of building up tons of muscle and knocking off tons of bodysize!

After about a month, soreness should stop being a problem, and you can just concentrate on walking faster and farther each day.

And speaking of "faster" and "farther:" take your time going for world-class mileages and speeds. A little ways into the program, you'll be walking distances and speeds that will **astound** you, so don't worry if you can't do them on Day One or Week One. They'll come. Just let your **body** tell you when, not the other way around.

Remember: you're here for one thing and one thing only: to get fit and lose bodysize.

As long as you walk as fast as you comfortably can for as long as you comfortably can every day, that's exactly what you'll do.

And when you do, you'll know how those athletes feel who stand on three-tiered platforms every four years— freshly-minted medals dangling from their necks—and watch, through tear-filled eyes, their countries' flags being raised, their national anthems filling the Universe.

Because that's exactly the way getting fit and trim will make you feel—especially if no one thought you could!

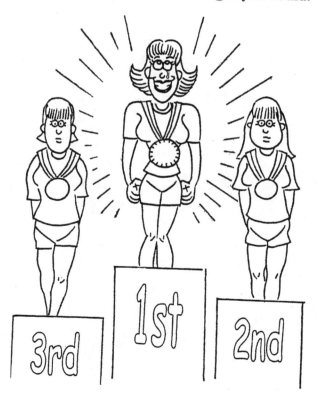

6

"Go Tell it to your Body"

One of the great miracles of life is that your body does exactly what you "tell" it to do.

When you Fitwalk, you're "telling" your body: "I'm going to be **using** these legs, so you'd better do whatever you can to **help** me use them!"

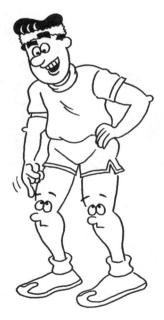

And your body does!

How?

By giving you the tools to walk farther and faster each time out:

Walking takes energy.

Your muscles get this energy from "power molecules" that they store.

As you Fitwalk, these molecules—which biologists call "glycogen" or animal starch—get used up.

When they're **all** used up, you've Fitwalked "as long as you comfortably can" and you might as well mosey on home—where you stand, with "empty" leg muscles.

And what does your body do when it "sees" that?

It starts replacing the glycogen.

But does it put back exactly what your Fitwalk took out?

No: it puts back **more** than your walk took out.

Why?

Because it **always assumes** you'll be walking even **farther** your next time out, and it has to give you the **extra fuel** to go those **extra miles**!

But that's not the only assumption the body makes:

Whenever you "challenge" your muscles, the way you do when you Fitwalk, there will always be a certain number of them that are not **up** to the challenge; these will break down.

When your body sees these broken muscles, it will sweep them away and build new ones in their place.

But does your body build new muscles that are the same size and strength as the old ones?

Not at all: it builds **bigger** and **stronger** muscles—and more of them!

Why?

Because it **always assumes** you'll need to walk even **faster** your next time out, and it has to provide the **extra strength** to go that **extra speed**!

Because of this "double 'overkill'"—putting back more power molecules than you took out, and building stronger muscles than you broke down—you find yourself with muscles that couldn't "drag" you five **feet** on Day **One,**

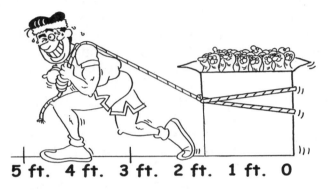

5 ft. 4 ft. 3 ft. 2 ft. 1 ft. 0

suddenly "whizzing" you five **miles** on Day **Twenty**-one!

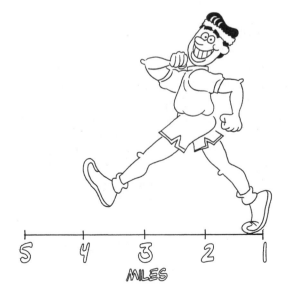

5   4   3   2   1
MILES

And all because you "told" your body that that's where you were headed!

The question, of course, is:
Where does all this new glycogen come from, and where does your body get the energy and raw materials to do all that muscle rebuilding?
The answer? Of course: from your fat pads:

1) After your walk, your body pulls some fat out of storage, changes it to glycogen and ships it off to its new home in the muscle, where it can fuel the rebuilding and your next walk.
2) Your body then pulls more fat out of storage, changes it into protein and uses that to make new muscle.

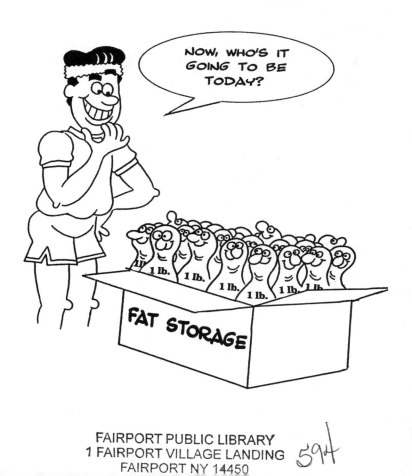

Which gives you the whole Fitwalking Story in a nutshell:

"Exercised muscles pulling fat from storage to 'recharge their batteries' and build themselves up!"

And how might that get you a little slimmer? Very easily: Since exercised muscles are slimmer than the fat they "pull,"

the more you exercise, the slimmer you get!

And all because of one simple thing: the fact that you got out there and "talked" to your body every day—one Fitwalking step after another!

"Details! Details!"

What is "Fitwalking?"

"Walking as fast as you comfortably can for as long as you comfortably can."

Good. And because of that, there are two things you should watch out for:

1) Because you're only walking as fast as you **comfortably** can, there's no need to time yourself: if your pace gets **too** comfortable, you speed up; if it starts getting **un**comfortable, you slow down. It doesn't really matter how fast you're going, because you're not trying to break any land speed records here.

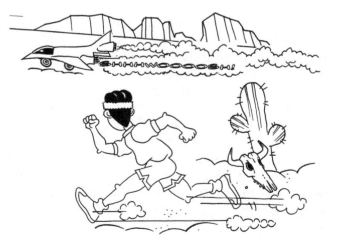

2) Because you're only walking as **long** as you comfortably can, there's no need to keep track of your mileage: you walk as long as you comfortably can and not a step further. Whatever the mileage is, it is, and **knowing** what it is won't add a single inch to the total!

The other way of going about it—worrying about "times" and "mileage"—can drive you crazy, because all of a sudden you've got daily targets to hit or you won't feel like you're making any progress.

And what happens if you don't hit those targets?

Well, what happens when most of us fall short of a goal? That's right: we get discouraged and depressed and try to eat our way back to happiness.

To keep that from happening, we ask you to forget about all **other** targets just this once and simply concentrate on **Fitwalking's** "target:" getting you fit and trim!

And how do you hit **that** target?   By doing nothing more each day than going out and walking as fast as you comfortably can for as long as you comfortably can. In other words, by letting your **body** tell you how well you're doing each day—not yesterday's performance charts!

And what will your body tell you each day?

Of course: that you're always doing **the best you can**, given the conditions of **that day:** weather; mental attitude; physical shape; and so on—and how much better can you do each day than "**the best you can**?!"

So don't be obsessed by "times" and "mileage."

Just Fitwalk every day and pretty soon you'll find out what every other Fitwalker has found out: that Fitwalking is a **joy**, and as long as you don't do anything that takes the joy **out** of Fitwalking—like worrying about "progress"—you'll want to do it forever. And stay **fit** forever!

If you can think of a **better** way to spend the rest of your time here, you've got our number!

8

"For the 'Progressoholic'"

Now where ya going?

"To get me one of those nifty 'sports' watches that lets me keep track of 'times' and 'mileage' and stuff."

But I just told you—

"Yeah, right. Hey: do me a favor——?"

What?

"—Work me up some kind of 'program' for when I get back with the watch?"

Oh. Sure.

Well, nobody else seems to listen when you tell them that curiosity killed the cat, so why should you?

Just promise us one thing: You want to keep track of your progress? Fine: go ahead. But we weren't kidding:

Your "progress" should be measured in things like resting heart rate, muscle tone, and, if you're real lucky, clothing size—not things like "lap times" or "total mileage". And, if becoming a "slave" to one keeps you from achieving the other, then you should take your "nifty 'sports' watch" and toss it into a nifty **river**!

Now that we've gotten that out of our system...

The best way to measure your progress from one day to the next is to walk a set circuit—what we call a "loop," which can be around your own neighborhood, a nearby park, a school running track, etc.

It doesn't matter how long this loop is, only that it's a fixed distance, so that you can compare your performance on it from one day to the next (a lot of folks have more than one of these loops, just for variety's sake.)

To get the distance for a residential loop, simply drive the loop and record its mileage.

If the loop isn't driveable—if it's in a park, for instance—then reverse the process: figure out how long it takes you to walk a mile at your normal speed (a school's running track is best for this), then time yourself around your undriveable loop at about that same speed. Then just divide the time around your new loop by your normal mile time and you'll get a rough idea how long your new loop is.

For example: if you know it takes you 16 minutes to walk a mile and you can get around your new loop in 12 minutes, then your new loop is about "12/16ths"—or "3/4"— of a mile.

The next step is to figure out how to use the sports watch (none of them is difficult to use; just work along with the instructions) and to start recording your "lap times," "total laps," "total time," "total mileage" (we've included a Walking Log with this book, to help you do all that.)

Just don't forget: your performance will vary from day to day, depending on a lot of things (weather; lung capacity; leg condition; companions; etc.), so don't expect your progress chart to look like a 747 taking off! In fact, a child's drawing of the Rocky Mountains may be more like it!

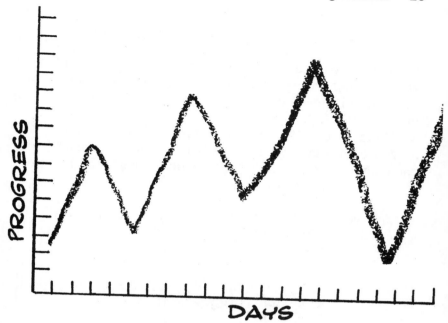

We'll say it again: Your best bet is to just go out every day and walk as fast as you comfortably can for as long as you comfortably can.

If you want to record your "lap times," etc., go ahead and record them; just don't be **obsessed** by them, and don't expect every day to be better than the one before it, because it probably won't be.

And, if you find that your "bad" days **are** making you discouraged, well...you know the way to the river!

The purpose of Fitwalking is to get you fit and trim and keep you fit and trim—not to make you want to shoot the cat because you won't be in the next Olympics (though as we've said: once you're a little ways into the program, you'll start chalking up speeds and distances that are impressive by anyone's standards. The only thing is: you may be walking those speeds and distances only every other day, or every third day, and unless you realize that and can accept it, you'll find yourself getting forever disappointed.)

So if you "can't live" without charting your progress, then do it.   But if you find yourself canceling Fitwalking sessions because you're afraid you won't be able to "perform" on a given day to the level you've been performing, then **stop** playing with your charts and get back to doing what Fitwalking is designed to do: get you **fit** and help you lose a little bodysize!

Which is exactly what will happen if you just walk as fast as you comfortably can for as long as you comfortably can each day—no matter how "fast" or how "long" that might be.

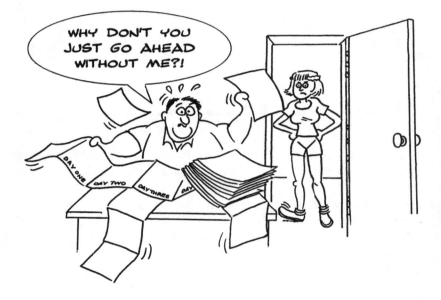

9

What to Expect

What should you expect from Fitwalking—especially if you're using it not only to get fit but to lose a little bodysize?

Well, we can tell you what **not** to expect—namely:

Don't expect to lose a ton of bodysize overnight!

We know that's the way you'd **like** it to happen (who wouldn't?), but it's not going to, so don't expect it.

In fact, real-world slimming—Fitwalking slimming—happens so gradually (in "ounces per day"), that you're better off if you

Don't expect to see ANY change in body size EVER!

Why?

Because nobody yet born can tell when the Pacific Ocean is "down a quart!"

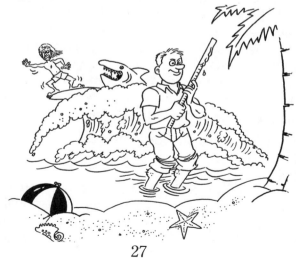

It's a little like the experiment where you blindfold someone and prick the skin over his thumb with a pin; then you move the pin a real small amount and ask him if it moved.

If you do it just right, he'll say "No," because our senses aren't fine enough to pick up on such small changes.

You keep going, moving the pin a little bit each time, and each time he says, "No, the pin didn't move."

When you're done, you tell him to take off the blindfold. And what he sees is the pin—that started at his **thumb** and that he said "never moved"—now sitting on his **shoulder**!

Which is the way Fitwalking works: you start out plus-sized and wind up **less** than plus-sized and you "never knew what hit you!"

So don't expect to. Because if you do, you'll find yourself getting disappointed.

So what?

Well what happens when most of us get disappointed?

That's right: we quit!

And try as we might, we've never been able to figure a way for Fitwalking to get you fit and trim if you're not doing it!

So do us a favor: Walk for any reason you can think of—

Walk because it's the "right thing to do;"
Walk because your heart and lungs will love you for it;
Walk because your legs will get "'goosey' gorgeous;"
Walk because it can ease the tensions of the day;
Walk because it "helps your hormones;"
Walk so that your kids will want to;
Walk because your life is better **with** a walking program in it than it could ever be **without** one;

—walk for any reason you want to, except one: to lose bodysize.

Why?

Because if you walk for that reason, you'll always be disappointed and you'll always give up, since you'll never lose as much bodysize per day as you'd like to be losing or think you should be losing; whereas, if you walk for any of those other reasons, you'll never get disappointed, because all those things are easy to achieve.

And what happens while you're reaching all those **other** goals? Of course: you'll "secretly" achieve the one you **really** want: getting a tiny bit slimmer every day.

We hate to make it look like you have to "sneak up" on slimness, but that's the way it works: expect Fitwalking to get you slim and it probably won't; expect it to do anything else and people will be admiring the New You from morning til night!

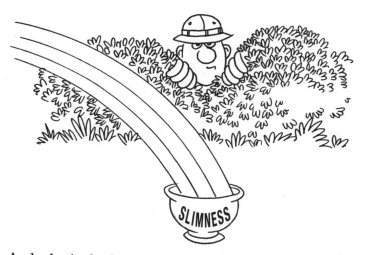

And what's the best way to get Fitwalking doing what you want it to do?

Easy: Just make it a normal part of your daily routine, along with all the other activities you don't have any special expectations for; things like brushing your teeth, taking a shower, shopping, eating, etc.

If you can do that—if you can make Fitwalking a normal part of your everyday life—then it will do everything you want it to do, including getting you fit and trim.

But if you can't—if you insist on making Fitwalking something it's not—the chances are real good that it won't do a thing for you!

And do you really need another one of **those** in your life?!

10

"Say Cheese!"

Of course, if you really want to see what Fitwalking is doing for you, there is a way:

Take pictures of yourself!

Specifically: have someone take your picture once a month from a variety of different angles: face-on; three-quarter front; side; three-quarter rear; rear. Wear as few clothes as modesty will allow, since we want to see changes in your **body**, not your wardrobe!

Take some of the photos with your arms at your sides, others with your arms in the air. Take some bust shots, some from the waist up, some full-body. Strike some poses, like the models do in magazines.

In this way—and only in this way—will you be able to see the progress everyone else has been seeing since the day you started Fitwalking.

One more thing about taking pictures: because slimming is go gradual with Fitwalking, not only won't you believe anything is happening while it's happening, you won't believe anything has happened once it's **done**!

That's why it's especially important to take pictures of yourself after you get down to your normal body size, because that's the only way you'll know how far you've come (you can't do it by looking at yourself in the mirror because you can't see all of yourself at once, like you can with a snapshot.)

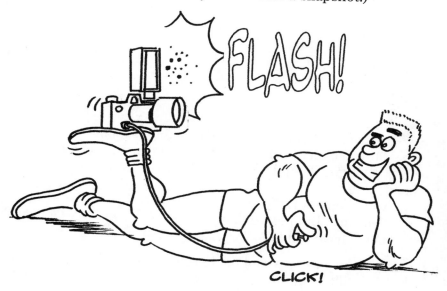

Unless you're made of stone, it won't take long for you to **fall in love** with what you see in those photos!

That's OK; don't be embarrassed! Let yourself go! Cry for joy, if you feel like it!

You've "reclaimed" yourself! Celebrate it!

And then take somebody **else's** picture!

11

"A Year to Go"

Quick review:
What's the only way that Fitwalking can fail?
"If you expect more from it than it can possibly deliver."
Very good! And what's the best way to keep that from happening?
"Get a lobotomy?"
Well, yes. But before that.
"Don't have a clue."

The best way we've found, to remove all fatal expectations from Fitwalking, is to tell yourself that, no matter how much bodysize you'd like to lose, you

Always have a year to go

to lose it:

If you're a hundred size-pounds overweight (see Appendix A), you have "a year to go" to get them off.
If you lose half those hundred, you still have "a year to go" to get rid of the other 50;
When you're only 10 size-pounds above your target body size, you still have "a year to go" to take those off;
And when you have only **one** size-pound left to lose, you still have "**a year to go**" to lose it!

Always having "a year to go" takes all the size-loss pressure off you, and lets you enjoy what Fitwalking is **really** doing for you, which is: beautifying your leg muscles and strengthening your heart, which will soon stop trying to pound its way out of your chest, every time you so much as roll over in bed!

Of course, in order to achieve its **primary** goals—beautifying your leg muscles and strengthening your heart—Fitwalking has to do one small thing: empty out all your fat stores. Which gives you a nifty little **side effect**, which we call: "Slimness!"

And to make sure you do get that side effect, just keep telling yourself, every time you look in the mirror and see a body that's a bit larger than you'd like it to be:

"No problem: I still have a year to go to get down to my target body size."

Until
one day
you do!

12

"Murphy's Law"

Your body pulls fat from its various storehouses in a built-in sequence. For one person, that sequence might be: "head-chest-neck-calves-etc.;" for another, it could be just the opposite.

However, no matter what our individual sequence might be, we all seem to be victims of our own special "Murphy's Law"—the original being: "If anything can go wrong, it will."

In the case of bodysize loss, our "Murphy's Law" reads:

"Wherever you really want the bodysize to leave, that's where it won't!"

For example: if you want your thighs to stay as plus-sized as possible, all you have to do is to wish with all your might that they'd get slim!

Day after Fitwalking day you'll stare at those thighs, and day after day the verdict will be the same: "No change!"

Everywhere else? "No problem:" your arms, shoulders, neck, chest will get as slim as it's possible to get, and do it in record time!

But those thighs? Forget about it!

And Heaven help you if you'd like some bodysize to come off your **waist**! We wish we had a dollar for everyone who lost 4-6 inches from his chest, 3-4 inches from each thigh, but not a **single millimeter** from his waistline while everything else was going "poof!"

In fact, if you're expecting to see any change at all in your waistline, expect it to look **bigger** before it looks smaller. Why? Because, as Einstein said: "Everything is relative:"

When you look at your waistline in a mirror, you judge how big it is by comparing it with structures around it, like your chest.

If your lower chest has gotten four inches smaller since you started Fitwalking, but your waistline only one, then your waistline will actually look like it's gotten three inches **bigger** since the day you began.

Which will, of course, do wonders for your spirits:

"What the heck's going on here?! I'm walking like there's no tomorrow, and all I'm getting is **bigger**?! Let me off this stupid 'bus!'"

And you'll start making plans for that hour you used to "waste" every day, trying to walk off a little bodysize.

And while you're making those plans, you'll slip on a pair of slacks that were tight last week, and you'll get ready for a real fight when you go to button them, since you're obviously larger than you were the last time you wore them.

Except...

When you do go to button them, you **don't** have to fight; in fact, the two sides come together rather easily.

At which point, you'll look at those slacks in the mirror and, when you've convinced yourself that they're the same ones you had on the week before, and that no one's snuck in and stretched them while you were out, your eyes will travel up from those slacks to look stunned at themselves:

"Ohmigod: it **does** work!"

And you'll get a cold feeling up and down your spine:

"What if I **had** gotten off the 'bus?' How much bodysize would I have **kept** myself from losing?!"

Answer: "All of it!"

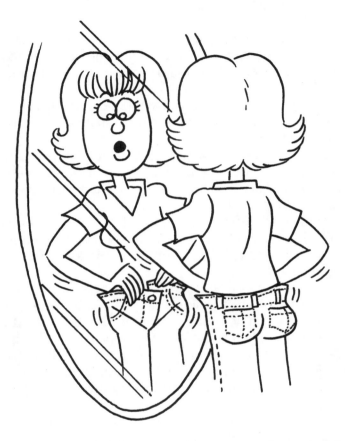

So don't ever leave the program because of what you **think** is happening. Remember: "seeing" isn't always "believing," especially in the case of your waistline, where you're forever seeing it next to other "structures," not next to what **it** looked like two weeks ago (which, again, is why **pictures** are so important.)

The fact is: **all** your bodysize will eventually go, and no one will ever care what order it went in.

The way it will happen is: once all the **non**-"Murphy" storehouses have been emptied of their bodysize, your body will turn its attention to the places **you've** been wanting it to leave for so long.

Suddenly, areas that couldn't lose "millimeters-per-month" will start dropping "inches-per-week," and you won't be able to update your wardrobe fast enough (do we have to tell you what a glorious day **that** is?!)

And if you didn't get a shudder before, you'll sure get one now:

"My God: What if I **had** given up on Fitwalking because it 'didn't work?' This day would never have come!"

That's right!

So don't risk that "day" by ignoring "Murphy's Law of Bodysize Loss" or "Einstein's Corollary."

Just keep Fitwalking every day and, in a few months, guess who'll be telling Murphy where **he** can get off!

13

A Word about Weighing Yourself

DON'T

14

Further Thoughts On Weighing Yourself

Though the last chapter was as complete as it needed to be (feel free to review it any time you want), we'd like to take a moment to expand on a few of its key points:

There are a lot of reasons you should never weigh yourself, on this or any other program:

1. There is nothing more meaningless than body **weight**; the only important thing is body **size**.

To show you what we mean:
Take your typical football tailback and the "couch potato" who watches him on TV every Sunday.
A likely height and weight for each of them would be 5'11" and 210 pounds.
If weight really meant anything, then both men would wear the same size clothes, get the same looks from the ladies, move with the same style and grace, etc.
And do they? Yeah, right!:
The tailback slips easily into Size 32 slacks, while the couch potato can only dream about getting into his 38's!

Women line up at the tailback's door, while the couch potato can't get a nod from his goldfish!

The tailback moves like a racehorse, while the couch potato sits and waits for the plow!

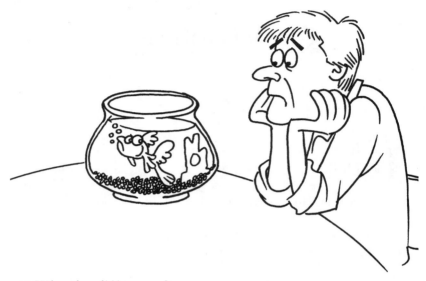

Why the difference?

Well, obviously: the tailback is 210 pounds of "muscle," the couch potato 210 pounds of "fat."

What does this tell us?

Simply that, on a **pound-for-pound** basis, "muscle" takes up a lot less space than "fat."

So if our couch potato could just "trade" every pound of billowy fat for a pound of lean, hard muscle, he could get a whole lot thinner without getting any lighter.

And can he make that "trade?" Of course he can: with Fitwalking. And so can you.

Since all you'll be doing, with Fitwalking, is "trading" pounds of bulging plus-size for pounds of lean, hard muscle, what sense would it make to weigh yourself? I mean, your **weight** may never change; only your **body size** will.

So don't do it, especially since weighing yourself can be such a "killer" (read on!)

2. The second reason for never weighing yourself is:

You don't know what you're weighing!

If you were weighing just body fat every time you stepped on a scale, and your weight went up or stayed the same after some serious dieting or exercise, then you could say for certain that that "diet" or that exercise didn't work.

But **are** you weighing just body fat? Or are you weighing everything **else** under the Sun: bones, muscles, organs, body fluids, gut contents?

Of course!

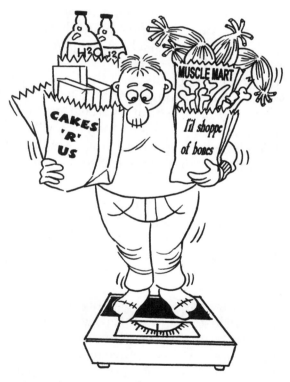

So when you step on a scale after dieting or exercise and the results are the exact opposite of what you were expecting, can you really say for sure that your weight-loss program didn't work (didn't eliminate fat)?

Or could your weight gain be due, for example, to some extra fluid your body retained, to process a load of salt (it takes **ten** water molecules to process **one** molecule of salt, you know)?

And what about food going in but not coming out (delayed bowel movement); you think three pounds of food isn't going to weigh three pounds, just because you can't see it anymore?!

The bottom line is: changes in weight can be due to a lot of things—not just fat loss—and unless you realize that, you will be facing terminal disappointment every time those changes don't go your way.

And what happens when someone or something disappoints you? Of course: if you're like most of us plus-sizers, you try to drown your disappointment in a hundred pounds of "goodies!"

No problem with that, except...

Later on, when you finally pass the fluid or food that was giving you those false readings and you realize you really **did** lose body fat on your "diet" or exercise program, it will be too late: the "hundred pounds of goodies" will again rule the roost, and you'll be back to where you started: pouring in the calories, but with no "diet" or exercise program to get rid of them for you.

To keep that from happening—to keep from giving up a bodysize-reduction program because you thought it wasn't working or was working in reverse—trust the fact that when you weigh yourself you have no idea what you're weighing. So, never do it, since doing it can be so disastrous!

3. Of the three things that weighing yourself can tell you—that you've lost weight, stayed the same, or gained a few pounds—all three can destroy your size-loss program.

We've just seen how destructive it could be if you expected to lose weight and either stayed the same or actually **gained** a little weight.

But what happens if you diet or exercise like crazy and actually **lose** weight? How could that be a "killer?"

Very easily:

Actually doing what you set out to do—in this case, "losing weight"—is always cause for celebration, isn't it? And how do you celebrate **everything**? Of course: if you're like most of us, with an extra-special **food** treat. And why shouldn't you, since your lovely weight loss has actually given you room to "cheat" a little.

Of course, when your mind and body once again get a taste of that "forbidden fruit", what are they going to do: not ask for more? Don't be silly! Give them one little hot fudge sundae and they'll be clamoring for another one. Then another one. Until that's **all** you're eating!

Nothing wrong with that, except the Walk Yourself Fit program tells you that, as long as you don't change what you eat, you **should lose bodysize**. In other words, if you had ten hot fudge sundaes last year, you can have ten hot fudge sundaes this year. But not ten hot fudge sundaes a **week**, because **nothing** could overcome that!

To keep that from happening—to avoid a "celebration" getting out of hand and destroying your get-fit program— never give yourself a **reason** to "celebrate."

In other words, **stay away from the scale**!

At one time, we weren't so insistent about people never weighing themselves. Then we heard of a woman who dropped four dress sizes by Fitwalking, got on a scale, discovered she hadn't lost any "weight" and immediately abandoned her Fitwalking program because it "didn't work"(?!)

Are we saying you'll be that silly? Of course not. But why risk it? Why give your Subconscious a chance to dub Fitwalking a failure, simply because it's confusing this **size**-loss program with all the other programs you've ever been on, which are based on **weight** loss?

To avoid being victimized by that confusion, we can't tell you strongly enough: get rid of your bathroom scale. Give it away, or hide it for a few centuries!

And then turn your attention to the **real** purpose of Fitwalking, which is to:

Get you fit;

Get you feeling even better about your body;

Get you into clothing sizes you always thought were for "other people."

And all you have to do, to get all this wonderfulness coming your way, is to go out every day and put in your miles.

Almost without realizing it, you'll start getting fitter—and maybe a little slimmer. Your step will be livelier, the air will smell sweeter, you'll begin **seeking out** your reflection for a change, instead of always going out of your way to **avoid** it!

Most important: you'll start **looking forward** to your Fitwalking sessions the way you **never** looked forward to day after day of "grapefruit-and-cottage cheese!"

And to make sure you don't jeopardize this wonderful new life of yours by falling victim to the evils lurking in your bathroom scale, we tell you one last time, and as fervently as our little hearts can muster:

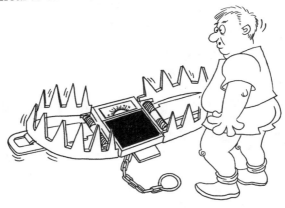

Never weigh yourself!

15

The Dawn of a 'New Age'

So, if you're going to get fit, and lose a little bodysize, you're going to have to control something: either the amount you eat or the amount you exercise.

"Right."

And which is easier: exercising more or eating less?

"Silly question!"

Do you know why?

"No."

Because every fiber of your mind and body has one goal and one goal only: to make sure you survive from one day to the next.

And, while **you** might call "half-a-grapefruit-and-black-coffee" a "diet," your mind and body call it "starvation." And since starvation is at all times a **threat** to your survival, your mind and body have no choice but to fight it, tooth-and-nail (think back to the last time you went on one of those things and you'll know just how "sharp" those "teeth" and "nails" can be!)

And how do the same mind and body feel about the other way to get fit: "exercise?"

Well, who do you think could flee a lion better: Fatty Arbuckle or Usain Bolt?

Exactly: when survival is on the line, the exercised body will always win out over the non-exercised one.

Your mind and body know this. Which is why, when you start to exercise, they fall all over themselves to help you: increasing blood flow to your muscles; building muscle at the expense of fat; driving you to exercise by making you "antsy" if you don't; etc.

So when you finally do decide to get fit, you have a choice: try doing it by dieting, and get nothing but a **fight** from body and soul, or do it by exercising, and get the undying **help** of those two guys.

Some choice!

Which is why we can say, without reservation:

THE AGE OF "DIETS" IS OVER!
THE AGE OF "FITWALKING" HAS BEGUN!

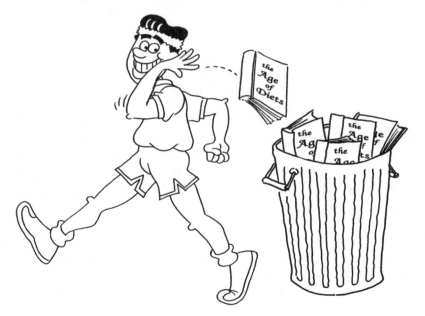

"But if exercise is such an odds-on choice for getting fit and trim, why are so many folks still trying to **diet** the bodysize off?"

For one simple reason: because they've been brought up to believe that exercise alone can't possibly burn enough calories to get the job done:

We all know the horror stories: you have to walk or run a whole **mile** to burn off the calories in a single pat of butter or an Oreo cookie! And, if those stories were true, the "experts" would be right: it would take forever to walk off all the butter and cookies in our lives!

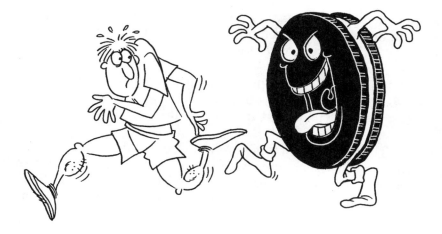

But those stories are not true:

Oh sure, you only burn about a hundred calories for every mile you walk or run. But those hundred calories are only what you burn **while you're walking** (or running)!

What happens after you stop? Does the calorie-burning stop as suddenly as your legs do? Of course not!:

When you walk briskly enough for your walking to be classed as "exercise," you break down a large number of muscle fibers. These broken fibers have to be swept away, and new ones built in their place. That takes energy, and lots of it!

Also, when you Fitwalk, you use up "power molecules" stored in your legs. Those molecules have to be replaced. **More** energy required!

So when all is said and done, you **haven't** burned just a hundred calories for every mile you've walked—you've burned **two** hundred or **three** hundred. And taken exercise from being an "impossible" way to lose bodysize to being a very effective way indeed!

Of course, an exercise like Fitwalking won't give you the pounds-per-day losses a good "starvation diet" will—at least for the first day or two of the "diet." But how many people do you know who've taken off bodysize on that kind of "diet" and kept it off? Or enjoyed doing it?!

Exactly!

And that figure is never going to change—**can't** change —because everything about a "diet" is "**anti**-survival," while every part of us is **just the opposite**!

Thankfully, with this new knowledge—that exercise alone can burn all the calories we need to, to get ourselves fitter and trimmer—we will never have to suffer the horrors of dieting again, but can go, instead, with a "sheer delight:" Fitwalking!

16

Why Fitwalking Works

OK, so the 200 calories I burn during a two-mile walk become 400 by the time you add in all the 'housekeeping' calories. So what? That still can't touch the four **thousand** calories I keep socking away every day!

"Even if I burn off 400, I'm still 3600 the 'wrong way,' so how can I possibly keep eating like that and still get fit?"

Very easily:

Let's say that you have, in fact, been averaging 4000 calories a day (and you're right: if you had to depend on exercise to burn them all off, the situation would be hopeless: you'd have to walk to Cleveland and back every day, just to "break even.")

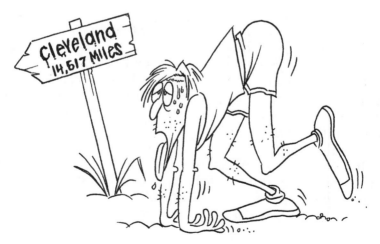

But let's see what's really been happening to those "four big ones:"

Say, for example, that you haven't been gaining more than 25 pounds a year (that's a hundred pounds every four years, so be careful before you protest that figure as being "too low.")

"Twenty-five pounds a year" is about "two pounds a month."

Since a pound of body fat contains about 3500 calories, that means you've been "gaining" about 7000 calories a month —or a little over 200 calories a day.

Get the picture:

Regardless what you've been eating every day, only **200 calories of it has been showing up as increased bodysize**!

How can that be, when you've been "packing away" those 4000 calories, day after day? Easy: your daily activities have been burning off the other 3800—which is not surprising, since it obviously takes more calories to move a heavy body around than it does a light one.

So, the bottom line is: you **don't** have to worry about the whole 4000 calories you've been scarfing down every day. All you have to worry about is the 200 **extra** calories that have been sneaking onto your waistline.

And how do you get rid of those extra 200?

Well, if one mile of Fitwalking will burn off a hundred calories while you're doing it and another hundred or so after you're through, you want to tell me what else you'd have to do, to hit that magic "200?"

"It's that simple?"

It's that simple: Walk one mile a day as fast as you comfortably can and you'll bring a guaranteed 25 pound-a-year weight gain to a **crashing halt**—without giving up so much as a single cookie!

And if someday you'd like to actually **lose** 25 pounds a year?

Well, how about walking **two** miles a day?!

Yes, we hear you:

"**Two miles**?!' I'm a hundred pounds overweight! Some days, I have trouble making it from one **room** to another!

"**Two miles**?!' Why not make it 'two **hundred**'! or 'two **thousand**!"

The reason we know where you're coming from is because we've just been there ourselves. And we know it's hard to believe, but you're going to have to trust us on this one: if you will just get started, walking as fast as you comfortably can for as long as you comfortably can every day, it shouldn't take you more than **two weeks** to get up to those two miles, no matter how plus-sized you were at the start and no matter how hard it might have been to put one foot in front of the other.

"Wait a minute: how can that be? How can everyone get to the same place in the same amount of time, no matter where each of them starts?"

We don't know; they just do!

It's a little like tearing a sheet of paper: no matter how big the original sheet, nobody you've ever met can manage the "seventh tear" (that is: you tear the original sheet in half, put the two halves on top of each other and tear those two in half, and keep doing that until you reach the "seventh tear.")

That "seventh tear" becomes the "great equalizer," making the strongest Goliath no mightier than the puniest David.

Which is exactly the way it works with Fitwalking: no matter how plus-sized you are at the start of those first two weeks, your leg muscles somehow build themselves up to the point where they can carry you two miles by the end of them.

So don't worry about "making the grade." Your body will give you all the tools you need, to Fitwalk as well as anybody your size ever has.

Just remember one thing: nobody ever got to the **seventh** tear without getting to the **first** (are you listening, little feet??)

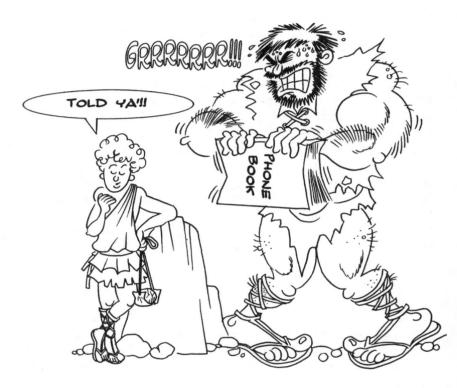

17

The Fly in the Ointment

Wait a minute! If all I'm 'putting on' is 200 calories a day, why can't I stop the size gain by cutting those 200 calories out of my diet? Or turn the **gain** into a **loss** by cutting out the whole **four** hundred?! Why do I have to **exercise** them away?"

Good question; easily answered:

The fact is, you **can** turn the gain into a loss by cutting down on what you eat—for a while. But eventually, this "diet" of yours stops working.

Why?

Because to keep losing size, your body has to keep pulling calories out of storage. The minute it stops pulling those calories out of storage, you stop losing bodysize.

And why would it stop?

Because the calories your body stores as fat are there for "Emergencies Only"—times of real famine, for example, which happened a million years ago and yesterday afternoon in Ethiopia—and, in the long run, anything that doesn't qualify as an "emergency" is just not going to get those calories.

"So what qualifies as an 'emergency?'"
Anything that threatens your survival:

Your body keeps you functioning on two levels: a Lower Level—"Survival"—and a Higher Level: "Thrival."

On the Survival Level, your body uses calories to keep your heart beating, your lungs working, and to keep everything else (muscles, brain, body cells) ticking along at minimum.

At the Thrival Level, your brain is able to engage in creative thought, your muscles have energy for long, hard workouts, etc.

If your body needs, say, 2000 calories to satisfy **both** levels, but you feed it only 1800, then you force it to make a choice: bring those "missing" 200 calories out of storage and keep everything functioning to the "max," or withhold those 200 calories from an "unnecessary"—i.e., Thrival Level— activity and "go with the 1800 we've got."

When you start your weight-loss program—a.k.a., "diet"— your body has "no problem" pulling those missing 200 calories out of storage to keep you "humming on all fours" (and giving you the nifty little size loss you were shooting for.)

However, as the shortfall goes on, day after day, your body does an about-face and starts thinking: "Hey: we've got 'starvation' happening here"—and it quickly "shifts gears:" suddenly, it stops "wasting" those stored calories on such "foolish" things as "solving problems" and "running a 10 K," and starts holding them back for more important things—like making sure you're **alive** next Tuesday!

So your 200-calorie cutback, which got you such a nice little size loss in the beginning, now gets you **nothing**.

So you cut back your eating by **four** hundred calories. But now your body is "on" to you and responds even quicker to your cutback with one of its own, so your size loss stops even sooner this time than it did before.

So you increase your cutback to **eight** hundred calories. And what does your body do? That's right: it finds a way to get along on **eight** hundred fewer calories, and every ounce of bodysize stays right where it was!

And on and on it goes, with your body matching your every cutback with an identical "hold-back" of its own, so the **less** you eat, the **less** fat it pulls out of storage and the **less** size you lose!

And what is the end result of all your body's "hold-backs?"

Well, since they all come at the expense of higher level functions, what you wind up becoming is a near-"zombie," mentally and physically: someone barely able to move, barely able to talk, barely able to think. In other words: someone of no value to his family, his employer, his customers—**anyone**!

And what's worse: someone not losing enough size to justify a **hundredth** of the torment he's going through!

Kind of cruel of your body to do that to you, especially when you're trying something as noble as losing bodysize. Unfortunately, your body isn't programmed for "noble;" it's programmed to keep you alive as long as it can, and, if you threaten that program by starving yourself, it'll be a cold day in you-know-where before your body bends over backwards to **help** you!

We would ask you to keep that in mind the next time some new-fangled "diet" comes along that promises it can get around your body's survival program. If it can, hey: go for it!

But if it can't—and there's only about a billion years of evolution standing in its way—you'd do well to think twice before mortgaging more than two or three of your children to go on it!

And while you're doing all this twice-thinking, you might get back to doing what evolution **wants** you to do and (here's a "sneak preview") **WILL release calories** for you to do: walking yourself fit!

18

Why Diets Don't Work

So how does your body feel about you going on a "diet?"
"Hates it!"
And what about your "other half"—that thing living inside your head? How do you think **it** takes to "dieting?"
"Like 'sunburn to sandpaper?'"
Well put!
"Thank you."
Do you know why?
"Same reason, probably."
That's right: "survival."

Do you know why you do everything you do?
"No."
Because a part of your brain called the Subconscious Mind **makes** you do it (the reason we call it the **Sub**conscious Mind is because it does all its work "behind the scenes" as it were, so we're not usually **conscious** of why it's making us do what we do; we just know that it is.)

Like the body, your Subconscious cares about only one thing: your survival. Do something to **threaten** that survival and your Subconscious Mind must stop you, and stop you **good**!

And what would threaten your survival? Well, how about a few months'-worth of cottage cheese-and-tomato slices?

"I can hardly wait."

Call that a "diet," do you?

"Who doesn't?"

Well, that's fine. But your Subconscious takes one look at that and thinks you've booked a flight to Somalia, and knows it "can't rest" until it's gotten you on the plane back home again. And the longer it takes you to get on that plane, the worse the trip becomes. Until, when you finally do "take off:"

"Gosh, Judy: I didn't know they **made** that many cookies!"

And when you've recovered from your cookie binge, you'll look at yourself in the mirror again and go running out to see what the latest tabloid has to offer:

"Gee," you'll tell your Subconscious, "this one sounds good: 'Papayas-and-Pork-Rinds! Lose a Million Pounds an Hour, Guaranteed!' So, what do you think, S. C.?"

Believe us: you don't want to know what your "S. C." thinks!

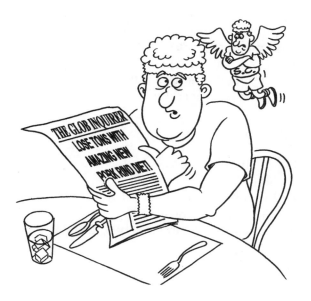

"O. K., I'll buy that: my Subconscious doesn't want me going off the deep end 'diet-wise'—especially 'diets' that are heavy into 'starvation.'

"But what about the other side of the coin—you know, when I'm 'packing away' everything in sight? Where's the old Subconscious then? If it's so interested in my 'survival,' why doesn't it stop me before my calorie count starts looking like the National Debt?!

"I mean, even **I** know the effect a zillion calories a day can have on the old life span!"

Exactly. So when your Subconscious lets you go through an all-you-can-eat buffet the way Sherman went through Georgia, it obviously has nothing to do with your **physical** survival.

"Then what else?"

The only thing left: **mental** survival.

"Wait a minute! You're telling me that 'five feet of fudge' is gonna keep me out of the Wacko Ward?"

Your Subconscious thinks it will.

"How?"

Well, what puts you **into** the Wacko Ward?

"Things that make me 'crazy!'"

And what makes you "crazy?"

"When I can't get a 'handle' on things."

Psychologists have a word for that.

"They do?"

Yes. They call it: "anxiety"—

"Oh."

—a feeling of "helplessness."

"Yeah, that's it!"

And what do you do when you get these feelings?

"Well, I go out and eat myself silly."

So you eat to relieve feelings of "helplessness."

"That's right"

Do you know why?

"No."

We might:

This "anxiety" we're talking about isn't exactly a new item in your life:

When you were a baby, and couldn't get a "handle" on things—when you felt helpless in the face of diaper rash or hunger or being left alone—you did the only thing you could do: you cried.

If you had a good Mommy—and most of us did—she heard your cries and came back into the room.

If you had, not only a good Mommy, but one who thought her "precious" was always about 20 or 30 seconds away from total starvation anyway, you got fed, no matter what it was you were crying about.

Unfortunately, what you were needing, a lot of the time, wasn't food, but just some reassurance that Mommy hadn't run off and joined the Space Program while you were in La-la Land. When you found out she hadn't, you stopped crying.

But did that stop Mommy? Not on your life! If your Mommy was like a lot of Mommies, she **knew** the Starvation Patrol was camped outside her door, just **itching** to drag her off to jail at the first sign of an undernourished child! So, like it or not, **YOU GOT FED**!

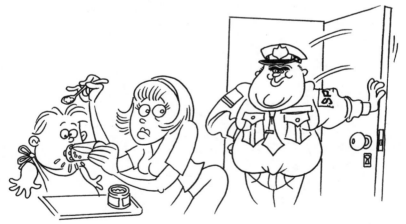

Years later, when a boss or a lover or a term paper is turning "La-la Land" into "Ca-ca County" and you could use a good dose of Mommy to "right your ship," there will always come a time when you can't **have** Mommy. Which will make you feel about as helpless as you did in that crib of yours.

What to do?

Well, you can't live very long, feeling helpless like that. Your Subconscious knows this, and, since its only purpose is to keep you alive, it knows it has to do something.

Do what?

Well, preferably, bring back Mommy.

But we know that's the one thing it can't do, so it has to come up with something else.

"What else?"

Well, what always went **along** with Mommy, every time she came back into the room?

"Mmm: yummy!"

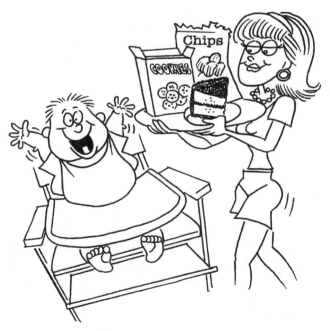

That's right: **food!**

So, as crazy as it might seem, every time you **want** Mommy but can't **have** Mommy, your Subconscious pushes you toward the next best thing: food!

And is it the "next best thing?"

Oh sure!:

No better way to get back on your boss's "A-list" than by "inhaling" five or six dozen cookies!

Want to lure your lover back into the nest? No problem: just drown yourself in hot fudge sundaes! That should do the trick!

And how about that term paper: why bust a gut doing research for it, when 15 or 20 Snickers bars can do it all for you?!

Right!

And the really sad part is, not only does the food not solve anything—after all, what could cold, dead candy bars do for you that the warmest, most **alive** creatures on Earth have trouble doing?—but that the foods your Subconscious gets you eating are almost always the kind you can't **stop** eating once you **start** (sugary; salty; buttery; etc.)

So not only does your Subconscious Mind's "solution" do nothing to relieve the **original** anxiety, it gives you a whole **new** anxiety to worry about: "plus-size," and the social rejection that often goes with it, no matter how much you wish it wouldn't or think it shouldn't.

And how does your Subconscious handle that new anxiety?

Of course: the same way it handled the old one: with more food!

Until you wind up doing nothing but you-know-what!

And what happens if you decide to "turn the tables" on your Subconscious—tell it you won't be "buying" its "solution" anymore; that you'll be going on a "diet" instead?

Well, think back to the **last** time you went on one of those things and try to remember what kind of "cooperation" your Subconscious gave you then (and they say pain has no memory! Right!)

So, what to do?

Easy:

Don't tell your Subconscious you won't be "buying" its "solution!" **Don't** go on a "diet!" **Don't** do anything that will make your Subconscious "get its back up!"

If it thinks you need a boatload of cookies to "survive," give it a boatload of cookies!* Don't keep forcing it to go overnight from a "boatload of cookies" to "grapefruit-and-cottage cheese," because it's never going to do it!

But, while you're giving in to its "cookie demands," never forget one thing:

The same Subconscious that needs you to eat has **absolutely no need for you to be plus-sized**!

That's right: as far as your Subconscious is concerned, as long as it gets you eating those cookies—and thereby "saving" you **mentally**—it could care less what those cookies are doing to you **physically**!

So what?

So take advantage of that "loophole." Eat every cookie your Subconscious wants you to eat, and then go out and walk them all off. **Your Subconscious won't stop you**!

And what will that do—eating cookies, then walking them off? Nothing much: just keep your Subconscious deliriously happy and out of your life, so you can work at making that life as deliriously happy as your Subconscious!

If, somewhere down the line, you can convince your Subconscious that it's been way off base all these years with its "food solution," fine: it can only make your Fitwalking that much easier.

But if you can't?

No problem: just keep walking!

So do it. Get off the couch, go out and get fit!

Don't spend a lot of time worrying about what you're eating or why you're eating it.

---

* Special health needs people, see Preface, pg. vii

If you **can** control your eating without tipping off your Subconscious, do it: it can only make your Fitwalking that much more effective.

But if you can't, **forget it**! Just go out and Fitwalk every day and you'll solve more problems then you ever thought you could!

19

"...from the Black Lagoon"

We're all creatures of habit:

Know of anyone who doesn't get hungry for the same breakfast/lunch/dinner/snacks at the same time every day?

And how about you smokers: look forward, do you, to making a phone call or starting your car without lighting up first?

And you "5:30 drinkers" out there: think it would be easy to simply "do without" one day, when "that time" rolls around? Yeah, right!

No: the list of things we do out of habit is virtually endless.

What's **not** so endless, though, is the list of reasons **why** we do them.

In fact, it stops at "one:" "survival."

"Wait a minute:"

What?

"You're telling me that the smoking driver **needs** to light up—to 'survive?!'"

Well, yes and no—

"—And that alcoholics have a better survival record than **non**-alcoholics?!"

Of course not—

"Then what exactly are you talking about here?"

I'm talking about what it **seems** we need, to survive.
"This better be good!"
Oh, it is:

Every day, two things happen:

1) You do a lot of stuff;
2) You make it to the next day.

What your Subconscious does is, it **connects** those two, thinking that the stuff you did was the **reason** you made it to the next day—not all that wacky an assumption to make, of course, since you did do both!

And, since its only job is to get you to Wednesday, how much simpler could things get:

If what you did on Monday got you to Tuesday, what better way to get you to Wednesday than by making you do those same things all over again—no matter how absurd or destructive those things might have been (and please note: your Subconscious makes no judgment about whether an action is "good" or "bad;" if you did it and survived, it thinks you **needed** to do it to survive, and it's going to **keep** getting you doing it over and over again until you tell it to stop!)?

And how does it get you doing the same things over and over again?

By setting off the physical "fireworks" (stomach churning; a "longing" in your gut; heart palpitations; etc.) that make you "hunger" to do those things, and drive you up a wall if you **don't**!

So, go ahead: have a jelly donut at 9:30 Monday morning and another one at 9:30 Tuesday, and see what happens to you, along about 9:30 on Wednesday.

That's right: you'll crave that jelly donut as if your life depended on it.

Why?

Because, to your Subconscious, **it does**!

So what?

So, if your life really **did** depend on that jelly donut, you'd be a fool to ignore your craving for it; that's called "starving yourself," and real starvation is at all times a bad thing.

But is starvation what's really going on here, or just what **seems** to be going on?

Obviously, if you're already carrying around 20, 50, 100 pounds more than you should be, then that case is closed!

Then why does it **feel** like you're always starving to death?

Because your Subconscious has access to the exact same "machinery" for making you hungry—and thereby getting you doing what **it** thinks you need to do, to "survive"—that your body has access to, to signal **real** hunger.

So what?

So, since you know that not satisfying real hungers will lead to starvation—which is at all times a bad thing—and since these hungers your Subconscious is creating for you seem as "real" as any your **body** has ever thrown your way, then the **last** thing you'll be doing is taking a chance that these real-**feeling** hungers might, in fact, be nothing of the sort.

Oh, no: you get a hunger, you're going to satisfy it, come Hell or high water!

Why?

Because to not satisfy it, you feel, is to risk certain death, and only a fool would do that!

And, since you're no fool, then **that** case is closed: Get hungry?—Eat! Case closed!

Which would be just fine, if all these hungers you were satisfying were, in fact, real hungers.

But again: how could they be, if your body already has weeks'-, months'-, or even years'-worth of food in storage?

Answer: they couldn't.

So what?

So, now that you know that nearly all of these hungers are phony ones—that you won't be starving yourself to death by ignoring a few of them every now and then—you can begin doing just that, starting today.

And what will that do for you: ignoring some of those hungers?

Well, in the same way you "train" your Subconscious to get you craving a jelly donut at 9:30 on Tuesday by **having** one at 9:30 on Monday, you can "train" your Subconscious to **stop** making you hungry for jelly donuts at 9:30 by **not** having them for a day or two!

And, as it happens: after you've put out the "fire below" by doing without something for a few days, you usually have trouble remembering why you thought that something was such a "life-or-death proposition" in the first place!

Do you **have** to put out the "fire below?"

No. As long as you walk off all those unnecessary jelly donuts, you'll still lose bodysize. It's just that it doesn't take a rocket scientist to see that if you **can** do without some of those extra calories, you can walk off your bodysize that much sooner.

And, if you do want to do without them, knowing that you only crave them out of **habit**, not out of any real **need**, should make your job that much easier.

So, if you would like to tackle your eating habits, to help your Fitwalking, you now have one of the most powerful tools on Earth for doing so: the knowledge that, no matter how "real" those every-five-minutes hunger pangs feel, they simply aren't; they're just a creation of your Subconscious Mind, to get you doing what it thinks you need to do, to survive.

And, if you'd rather not tackle those eating habits; if you'd rather not take the chance that all those hunger pangs are phony?

No problem: just keep walking!

And who knows: if you Fitwalk at 5:30 today and again at 5:30 tomorrow and then 5:30 the next day, maybe your Subconscious will do for Fitwalking what it so easily does for donuts and beer: turn it into a _____!

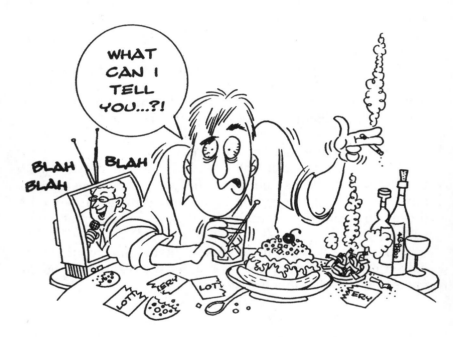

20

Wrapping it Up

So now you have the whole picture:

• When you could use a little human companionship but can't get it, your Subconscious Mind pushes you toward the "next best thing:" food.

• The food doesn't solve the problem—in fact, makes it worse—but it's the only "solution" your Subconscious Mind has, so it keeps pushing it on you.

• Most of the foods your Subconscious gets you eating are chemically addictive—sugary; salty; buttery—so you **keep** eating them, long after the psychological reasons for doing so have vanished.

• Your Subconscious remembers what you ate yesterday and notices that you survived to today. It then "connects" those two events and thinks that all it has to do, to get you to tomorrow, is make you eat, today, exactly what you ate yesterday. Until eating that way becomes impossible **not** to do; becomes, in other words: a "habit."

Breaking this incredibly complex eating cycle—which is what all "diets" try to do—is a monumental task, and one that is better left for another time and place, especially since we don't **need** to break it, to get fit and lose bodysize.

For now, just keep it in the back of your mind as you "suggest" to your Subconscious that it make your daily **Fitwalk** an "impossible thing not to do;" something along the lines of....that's right: a "habit!"

21

The Magic of Fitwalking

So how does your Subconscious feel about "dieting"?
"Hates it!"
–and your body?
"Same way!"
You know why?
"I'm wai-i-iting..."

Your body's main function, for the last 20 million years or so, has been to get you to distant hunting grounds, where you can run after a buffalo, kill the buffalo, then somehow get the buffalo back to your cave.

That you now need a computer to even **spell** "buffalo" is irrelevant: as far as your body is concerned, you could be hunting the big guys tomorrow and it has to be ready for you, in the same way your great-great-...-great grandfather's body was "ready."

And what does it mean to "be ready?"

Well, first of all, it means that your body has chosen fat for storing most of its energy, rather than the starch that plants use, because, at 9 calories of energy per gram of fat—vs. the 4 of starch—you more than double your chances of getting to the hunting grounds and back.

Second, it means that your body is programmed to **conserve** your fat stores when something threatens them, since it has to be sure it can always "buy" you that round-trip ticket to Buffaloville.

Nothing wrong with all that—after all, it's the reason you're here to read these words—except when you go on a "diet." Then, you wish your body had never **heard** of a buffalo:

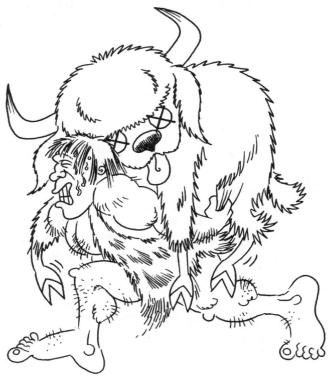

What was a good thing—fat being able to squeeze so many calories into such a tiny space—now becomes a bad thing, since you have to deny yourself an "ocean" of calories to get rid of a "teacup" of fat.

And that's just for the **first** "teacup!"

By the time you're going for Teacup Number Two, your body has already shifted into "Conservation Overdrive" and you have to turn your back on **two** oceans of calories to get the same results. Then **three** oceans; then **four**. Until you wind up doing without a whole **world**ful of calories to get rid of a "thimbleful" of blubber!

And what does your life look like, along about "thimble time?"

Just great: you're weak as a kitten, irritable as Scrooge, trying to remember how your shoes are tied, and looking like you're doing an all-day "step test" with your bathroom scale, hoping the darn thing will register **something** that'll make it all worthwhile!

When it doesn't, you throw up your hands and come down with an ice cream cone in each one, instantly whisking your mind and body out of Dieter's Hell and back into Non-Dieter's Heaven!

Where you stay.

Until the next "miracle diet" comes along that wonders why you're worrying about something as silly as a billion years'-worth of evolution!

At which point, it's "off to the races" again!

Of course, there's really no need to **fight** evolution when you're trying to get fit and lose bodysize, because it's so easy to get evolution's **help**.

How?

By doing so in a way where you work **with** Nature for a change, rather than **against** her: by **using** calories, rather than **restricting** them.

In other words: by **exercising**, rather than by **dieting**.

And why is it that your body views exercising as such a Godsend? Because exercised muscles are survival muscles, and your body loves the sound of that word!

And how does your body show its love?

In a remarkable way: the same body that so zealously **guarded** its stored calories when using them would **threaten** your survival, now sends them forth **gladly**, since it knows that doing so will greatly **increase** your chances of making it through.

And what is the end result of all this sending forth?
Of course: easy and permanent fitness and bodysize loss.

Which is what gives Fitwalking a power, a magic, that no "diet" could ever possess:

Every time you Fitwalk, you break down a unit's-worth of muscle. Your body then releases a unit's-worth of fat to help rebuild that muscle. This makes you one unit **stronger** on Day Two than you were on Day One.

Every time you Fitwalk, your leg muscles use up a unit's-worth of "power molecules" to fuel your walk. Your body then releases another unit of fat to replace those power molecules, which makes you one unit **lighter** on Day Two than you were on Day One.

Get the picture?:
Every "unit" you walk uses up **two** "units" of fat;
Every "unit" you walk makes you one unit stronger and one unit lighter, so you can walk **one unit faster and one unit farther** on Day Two than you could on Day One!

In other words: everywhere you look, Fitwalking is giving you a **two-for-one exchange**!

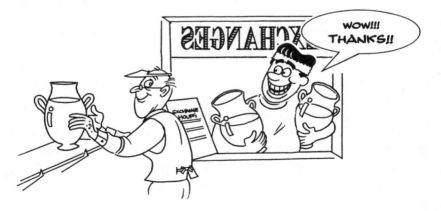

And what sort of "exchange" does a "diet" give you?

Well, when you deny your body a unit's-worth of calories, the most it can do is burn a unit's-worth of stored fat to make up the difference. That's it: no new muscle, no power molecule replacement—nothing! Just a "one-for-one" exchange—and then, only if you're real lucky!

And because of the way it works, not only is Fitwalking a more **efficient** way to lose bodysize than "dieting" could ever be, it also has the wonderful "side effect" of making you look **forward** to each lost inch—not cringe at the thought of what it's going to take to lose it.

And one more thing: when you lose bodysize by dieting, all you're doing is emptying out your fat stores. So, when an extra calorie sneaks into your body—and it will—it has only one place to go: those same fat stores.

On the other hand, when you **walk** off bodysize, you build these highly-efficient "metabolic furnaces" in your legs, known as "muscles." Now, when that extra calorie gets past your watchful eye, it has a **choice** of places to go to: it can get stored in a fat pad, like before, or it can get burned in the new muscle and vanish forever!

"So is that what Fitwalking guarantees—that none of those extra calories will ever turn to fat?"

No. Fitwalking just gives them a **chance** not to be turned to fat—which is a lot more than they got on your "diet."

So your choice is clear: try to lose bodysize by dieting, and watch yourself get weaker and meaner each day, with every extra calorie you eat turning to fat. Or **walk** the bodysize off, and watch yourself grow stronger and more alive, as your body grows smaller and smaller, while you at least give all those extra calories a **chance** to get burned, rather than stored.

As we've said before: some choice!

Which is why we can again proclaim it:

THE AGE OF "DIETS" IS OVER!
THE AGE OF "FITWALKING" HAS BEGUN!

—and welcome you to that magical New Age!

22

Control

How do you feel about self-control?

"Hate it!"

Much more fun to be **out** of control, isn't it: smoking and drinking and eating everything in sight?

"Absolutely!"

But you'd still like to get fit and trim, right?

"Why do you think I'm here?"

So, you don't want to control yourself—

"Right."

—but you do want to get fit and lose a little bodysize?

"Also right."

And you really think you can do one without the other?

"I don't know, but I'll probably die trying!"

Well, maybe we can stop you a few steps short of the grave:

First of all, it really is a fact of life: if you're going to get fit and lose bodysize, you're going to have to control **something**! If you don't want to control the amount you eat, then you're going to have to control the amount you exercise. There's no getting around it.

"Oh, poop!"

But all is not lost.

"It's not?"

No. Because when you finally stop trying to "diet" the bodysize off and turn to exercise instead, you hit the "mother lode:" instead of having to control yourself **24** hours a day, which is what you have to do on every "diet" you've ever been on, all you have to do is **trade** one of those eating hours for an hour of Fitwalking, to get the same or better results!

What you do with the other 23 hours is your own business, as long as you don't eat **more** than you normally would!

If you can do that—if you can "control" yourself that one hour a day—you can do whatever you want (within obvious limits) the other 23, and still get as fit—and lose as much bodysize—as you'd like.

So, do it!

23

"The Best Thing"

If there's one thing we all need, it's achievements; without them, we're little more than plant life. Unfortunately, most of us are so busy earning a living in a routine way that we don't get many chances to pile up such achievements. Which is where Fitwalking comes in:

No matter how bad or insignificant our day may otherwise have been, Fitwalking is always there to make sure we have at least one shining moment we can point to; something we can rely on to make us better off today than we were yesterday: more fit/less plus-sized; happier; more alive!

It is this sense of **achievement** that sets Fitwalking apart from every other size-loss program—this feeling that you are, in **every** way, a better person today than you were yesterday, and that you've gotten there by doing something **positive** for yourself—Fitwalking—rather than something **negative**: "starvation."

Which is why Fitwalking is an almost-impossible habit to break, why Fitwalkers would rather give up **anything** than their daily fitwalk:

Today they walk six miles; tomorrow they'll shoot for seven!

When they started, they could barely move; now they're a blur!

Before fitwalking, their lives could be miserable; now they're a joy!

And the nicest thing about these "miracles" is that they're so easily gotten: all you have to do is put one foot in front of the other each day, as fast as you comfortably can for as long as you comfortably can.

Of course, if you have something better to do during that hour-or-so, something that will make your spirits soar just as high, far be it from us to take you away from that.

But if you don't—if you could use an extra dose of accomplishment—why not join us on the street, in the park, at the track?

We'd love to have you!

And you know something: so would you!

24

"...and twice on Sundays!"

You say I should Fitwalk every day."

That's right.

"But some days, I can barely move. Am I really doing myself any good, dragging my butt around the neighborhood for all of five minutes?!"

Physically, no. But otherwise, yes:

Your goal, for anything good you do, should be to make it a habit.

Why?

So you just do it automatically, which guarantees it will get done.

And how do you make something a habit?

Just one way: by doing it over and over again.

Which is why you should go for a Fitwalk every day, even if they need a time-lapse camera to tell if you're moving!

And one other reason: as we've already said: you often don't know, at the start of a walk, how good you'll be feeling five or ten minutes into it. And if you don't give it a shot, you'll **never** know.

So that's why you should at least **try** to walk every day.

If, after giving it your all for those five or ten minutes, you really don't have it, then quit; things aren't going to get any better and you're only fooling yourself if you think they will.

Remember, there's always "tomorrow." Just make sure "tomorrow" really **is** "tomorrow," and not "today."

To do that, test it; try to walk. If it's "not there," it's "not there." But at least try!

Every day!

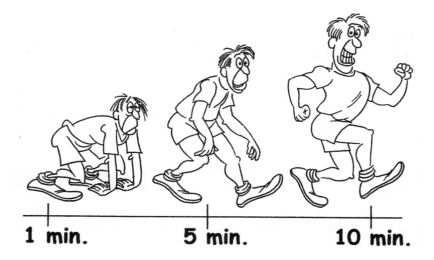

1 min.   **5 min.**   **10 min.**

25

"To Your Health!"

Was that your bumper sticker we saw?
"Which one?"

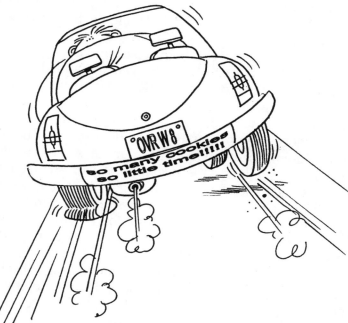

"Yeah, that's mine! You like it?!"

Real cute! And we were going to talk to you about "health!"

"So—talk away!"

But—

"Look: I love my cookies. But I've been thinking..."

Yes?

"You know those life-expectancy charts you sent me?"

From the insurance company?

"Right. Well, I finally got around to looking at them last night, and they got me thinking..."

Yes?

"Maybe those cookies **aren't** my 'best friend.' Maybe I **could** use a change."

We've all seen those charts. What they tell us is that, all else being equal, normal-sized people tend to live a lot longer than plus-sized ones.

But what those charts **don't** tell you is: all else being equal, **fit** people tend to live a lot longer than **anybody**!

So what?

So, no matter what body size you might currently be, you're always better off if you can get that body as **fit** as possible—and maybe lose a little bodysize in the process.

And why is exercise a better way to lose that bodysize than dieting could ever be.

Because, when you try dieting away the bodysize, all you're doing is emptying out your fat stores; you're doing nothing to challenge the organs that can give you a longer, healthier life: your heart, your lungs, your blood vessels, etc.

On the other hand, when you **walk** the bodysize off, you get those health-builders working for you from the very first step, so that, by the time you're down to your proper body size, that body is not just "unfat"—it's **fit**!

Which means you get a double bonus from Fitwalking: not only is it an **easier** way to lose bodysize than dieting (you're not fighting your Subconscious Mind all the time), but you're also **healthier when you get there**!

Of course, all you really have to do, to make up your mind about which way to go—dieting versus exercise—is look at the **glorious** face of someone who's **walked** the bodysize off, and compare it to the **death-warmed-over** face of someone who's tried to do the same thing by dieting! The minute you do that, there'll be only one thing left to say:

"Welcome to the World of Fitwalking!"

26

Christmas

With the Walk Yourself Fit program, every day is "Christmas," especially if you've been able to add a bit of reduced eating to your Fitwalking:

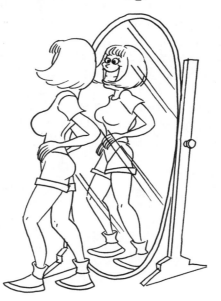

You can't wait to get up in the morning and put your clothes on, to see if they might be a little looser today than they were the day before (remember: you'll never be able to

see any change in body size from one day to the next, so don't expect to.)

You admire yourself from as many angles as you can; you can't get enough of yourself.

That's OK: don't be embarrassed by it. You deserve it. You've earned it. It's normal.

One piece of advice, though: always save the clothing you were wearing when you started the Fitwalking program.

Why?

Because, as you keep looking at yourself each "every-day-is-Christmas" morning, you may seem to get bigger and bigger before your very eyes, until, after a few minutes of looking, you decide that there has, in fact, been no change from the day before, and you start feeling disappointed—forgetting, of course, that we've told you all along that you may never **see** any change from one day to the next.

If this does happen to you, just go to your closet and haul out those extra-large clothes you were barely getting into when you began Fitwalking. Put them on. **Now** look at yourself.

If seeing the overall progress you've made since the day you began doesn't wipe away all of your disappointment, then I don't know what will.

Trust us: it will.

And you can just relax and go back to enjoying "Christmas morning!"

27

For the Few

When I was in junior high school, I had a friend—Stan —who had as perfect a physique as you could possibly have (eventually, Stan "used" this physique to become a champion long-distance runner.)

I, on the other hand, had the worst body in the history of the school—50-60 pounds overweight at all times—and the only physical activity I ever got was lighting up as many cigarettes as I could steal from my mother's purse!

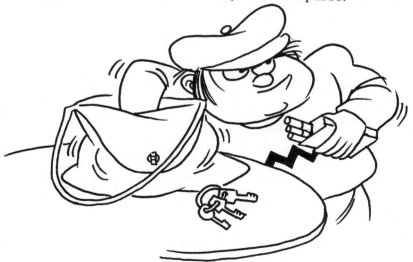

How Stan and I got to be friends I'll never know, except that a lot of mothers would tell their sons: "Go hang out with Rives! He may be a degenerate slob, but he's also very bright, and it wouldn't hurt your report card any if a little of that 'brightness' rubbed off on you!"—and I've got a feeling that's what was going on here.

Anyway, not only did Stan and I have different bodies, we had different **attitudes** toward our bodies:

Whereas I saw nothing wrong with the way I looked and couldn't wait for lunch (where I'd race through my own meal, so I'd have time to polish off everyone else's), Stan was always on a "diet:" starving himself the minute he could pinch a microscopic bit of fat around his middle (I tried to tell him that what he was pinching was what most people called "skin," but he wouldn't hear of it!)

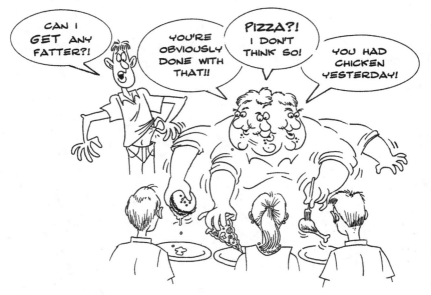

The upshot of the story is that Fat David kept getting fatter and fatter, while Skinny Stan never gained an ounce his entire life.

Why bring that up here?

For one reason:

This book was written to help historically plus-sized people—people like myself. And yet, I have a pretty good idea who'll be buying it and getting the most benefit from it: the "Stans" of this world: folks who woke up one morning and suddenly found themselves 10, 20 pounds overweight, and now "can't rest" til they've gotten rid of them!

However, if you're one of those plus-sized people, and you happened to come across this book and think you might like to use it to **join** the "Stans" of this world, we dedicate this chapter to you.

Having recently been a nifty 100 pounds plus-sized myself, I know what you're up against when someone says, "Go—walk yourself fit:" at that size, I couldn't walk five **feet**, never mind "**fit!**" In fact, if someone had asked me if I had any working muscles in those tree trunks hanging from my hips, I would have wondered what planet he was from!

And yet, even though I could barely move, I knew that Fitwalking held the answer to all my prayers: getting fit and losing bodysize without giving up any of the foods I lived for.

So, off I went, to "walk myself fit."

And how did I do the first day?

You got it: I walked five feet—and did it in well under a minute!

The second day I did much better: ten feet (unfortunately, I left my watch at home, so I don't know how long it took me. About a minute, I reckon, but definitely less than two.)

The third day, I managed what seemed like 50 or 60 feet—to the end of my block and back. Of course, that stretch is slightly uphill, so it was the same as if I'd walked a **hundred** feet on level ground (marathoners of the world: look out!)

Anyway, there I was: Three days into the program and still going nowhere.

So, what finally happened?

Well, to make a long story short:

Two weeks later, I was coasting my way through two **miles** (that's right: "**miles!**");

A week after that, I managed to do four miles in under an hour (not "**incredibly** under;" just "under!");

Another two weeks and I was doing five miles in that same hour!

The point is: what if I had given up after that first day? or the second? or the third? Where would I be now, except the obvious: 100 pounds plus-sized?

Where I would be is: someone in the same old rut, doing nothing to get himself out of that rut.

The question is: Is that really any way to live—to be doing nothing to make your life better—especially when something like Fitwalking can do it so easily?

So my advice to you historically plus-sized people is:

1) Get started
2) Don't quit.

I don't care if you only do the same five feet I did on Day One. As long as you do those five feet as fast as you comfortably can, you'll be Fitwalking: you'll be using some power molecules in your legs—which will have to be replaced—and you'll be tearing down some muscle fibers— which will have to be rebuilt. And to do both those things, your body will have to take fat from wherever it's stored.

And every time the power molecules get replaced and the muscles get rebuilt, you'll be able to walk faster and faster and farther and farther, until you're walking distances and speeds you thought I was joking about!

All you have to do is get started. Don't worry how far or how fast you're going. Just get out and Fitwalk every day.

Soon, you'll forget how painful it was to move those first five feet. Soon, you'll realize you **do** have muscles inside those "tree trunks," and they feel **good** when you use them!

By the way, if they **don't** happen to feel good on a particular day, that's because the power molecules **haven't** all been replaced and the muscle fibers **haven't** all been rebuilt. I mean, just because you **want** them to be doesn't mean they **will** be—especially if you're in your "middle years."

Not to worry: just walk as fast and as far as your "healing" legs will take you. The next day—or the one after that—will find you bounding around like a gazelle again, so who cares what happened the day before?

And soon after you've started your Fitwalking program, you may wake up to find your clothes "falling off you." At which point, you'll simply have "no choice" but to go out and buy new ones.

And you'll be very nonchalant around the salesperson, and with all the people you meet on the way home, where you'll slam the door behind you, "leap" into your new clothes, and dash to the mirror to see how you look!

Which will be: "Terrific!"

And the week after that? "**More** terrific!"

And the week after that? "So good I can't **stand** it!"

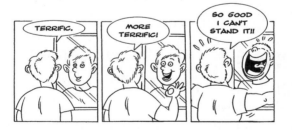

It's all possible and it's all so easy.

All you have to do is get started and your dreams of getting fit and losing bodysize will finally come true.

Take it from me, who used to be you.

28

Going on a "Diet"

So you know how senseless it is to go on a "diet."

"Absolutely!"

So what will you most likely do, sometime during the next year?

"Go on a 'diet.'"

Why?

"Because I'm plus-sized?"

No, because you believe in magic.

And since that's what most "diets" promise—

"Lose 10 Pounds in 5 Minutes!"

—they're right up your alley.

Unfortunately, you probably **will** lose ten pounds in five minutes!

"I will?!"

Yes—all of it "water."

But that won't matter: you'll step off the scale thinking you've finally arrived in "diet Heaven" (forgetting, of course, that those are the exact same results that all the "diets from Hell" ever gave you!)

And you'll order a new wardrobe, and cancel your life insurance, and begin making all sorts of plans for the Wonderful New You.

Until, of course, the magic "goes south" in the **second** five minutes and you never lose another ounce!

What went wrong?

Nothing. You just read the headline wrong. You thought it said: "Lose 10 Pounds **Every** 5 Minutes!"

Since that's impossible—we humans wouldn't have lasted this long if fat were that easy to lose—you're right back where you started: slogging your guts out to drop an ounce or two a week.

Before you go on your next "slog," try this:

Think of your plus-size as a redwood tree that you're trying to chop down.

There are two ways to chop down any tree:

- An inch at a time
- With one mighty blow.

If I were the tree, and I knew that the only way you'd consider me properly felled is with one mighty blow, I'd be real happy about things, since I'd know that what you were asking would require something called "magic," and there "ain't no such thing!"

On the other hand, if you had a sudden change of heart and could live with chopping me down an inch at a time, I'd know my goose was cooked, since my only defense against you—that there is no such thing as "magic"—would now be completely useless.

When it comes to chopping down your personal "redwood" (losing bodysize), Fitwalking is of the "one-inch-at-a-time" school; everything else—"miracle diets," fasting programs, etc.—are of the "one-fell-swoop" variety, and you'd do real well to stick a rabbit up your sleeve before going on your next one!

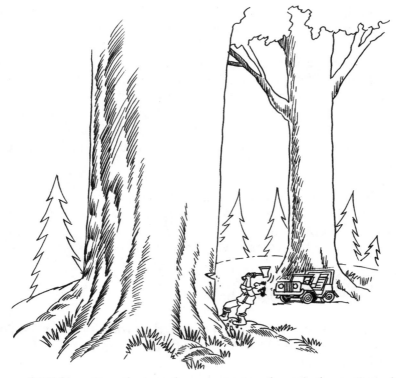

Will knowing that such programs rely strictly on "magic" get you to stop pursuing them! Of course not:

Has telling people that the odds against winning the lottery are 100-million-to-one ever stopped anyone from playing it? Not on your life!:

As far as we're concerned, there's a "magical" way that impossible things can become possible and we'll never stop searching for it.

Fine! Search for it!

But while your "magical" self keeps bouncing off your "redwood," no matter how promising an "axe" it might use, you might try slipping your **non**-magical self a cute little "hatchet" called "Fitwalking" every day, and letting it whittle your "tree" down an inch at a time.

That way, it won't matter if your magical "axe" never comes through: your "tree" will be gone and you can **tell** people it did!

So do us that one favor: while you're waiting around for some "magic" to come along, don't pass up the guaranteed results that Fitwalking can provide, as "unmagical" as those might seem.

And when you do decide to "go for the 'magic,'" never forget that it's virtually impossible to lose bodysize by "miracle" programs alone—since they're all based on varying degrees of starvation, and the **more** you starve your body, the **less** fat it brings out of storage; meaning that the only hope your "**diet**" has of getting rid of bodysize, after the first day or two, is whatever **exercise** you're doing with it.

A word of warning, though: if your new "diet" makes you so weak or discouraged that you want to give up on **all** size-reduction programs—Fitwalking included—abandon that "diet" immediately, so you won't be throwing out a very healthy "baby" (Fitwalking) with some very sorry "bathwater!"

Aside from that: "diet" away! See if you really **can** live on papayas-and-prune juice the rest of your life. Maybe there **is** some weight-loss magic in paying twenty dollars for a dead fig, or going without solid food for a couple of decades, or "exchanging" a piece of cheese for two apples!

But while you're jumping from one screwball program to another, never forget one thing: Fitwalking, all by itself, will enable you to lose all the bodysize you want, and do it the way Nature intended. It may take what you consider a long time—1-2 years, depending on how plus-sized you are—but after all: that size went **on** an ounce at a time, so what could be more "natural" than to take it **off** the same way?

Some people, of course, prefer that "guaranteed ounce" to a "pipedream pound."

Those people are called Fitwalkers and Fitwalkers don't believe in magic.

Hopefully, neither do you!

29

"If you can..."

Why is Fitwalking so successful?
"Because you don't have to change the way you eat."
Good. But what if you **could** change the way you eat?
"Then I guess you'd be even **better** off!"
Exactly: fitwalking burns fat, and the less new fat you create, the more old fat it can burn.
"Makes sense."
Luckily, if you decide you do want to change the way you eat, there are a lot of easy ways to do it:
"Like...?"
Well: How do you feel about "wasting food?"
"Hate it!"
A crime, is it?
"Of the worst kind!"
How about: "cleaning your plate?"
"Makes me think of Mother Teresa."
That good, huh?
"Oh, definitely!"
Gives you kind of a warm glow, does it?
"All over!"

Good. And what kind of glow do you think it **would** give you if it weren't **total nonsense**?

"Excuse me?!"

That's right!

"Get outta here!"

And not just **harmless** nonsense! Oh no: it's a good bet that more lives have been ruined around this little bit of nonsense than around any other nonsense in human history.

"But everyone knows—"

You're right: "everyone knows." So nobody "questions." Except one person:

"Who?"

A Dr. Joyce Bockar.

"Who's that?"

She wrote a book a few years back: *The Last Best Diet Book*. Finally blew the lid off this "wasting food/cleaning your plate" insanity.

"How so?"

By proving that there **is** no such thing as "wasting food" and there **is** no virtue in "cleaning your plate:"

First of all: once you turn a cow into a hamburger, it can never again become a cow. So if anything was "wasted," it was "wasted" long before **you** got hold of it!

And no matter what you do—eat the burger or throw it away—you can't "unwaste" the cow. So why keep trying?

To **"honor"** the cow, perhaps? To thank her for giving up her life so you could have a Big Mac?

Well, nice thought. But better to "honor" a waistline that **can** be changed than a cow that can't!

"But what about all the people starving in Ethiopia?"

What about them?

"Well, shouldn't you clean your plate because of them?"

Oh, absolutely!

"See?"

And after you've cleaned one plate for the Ethiopians, why not clean another one that you don't want or need for their Somali neighbors?

"I could do that."

And while you're sitting there, digesting all that food, could you do us a favor:

"What?"

Try to figure out what effect "'cleaning your plate' in Des Moines" could possibly have on **anyone** starving **anywhere**!

"Well-l-l..."

Take your time: you'll need all you've got!

Why we fall for this nonsense—have **always** fallen for it—is beyond me.

Do you think those starving Ethiopians and Somalis are all huddled around a Western Union office somewhere, waiting for news of how much food you're finishing in Iowa...

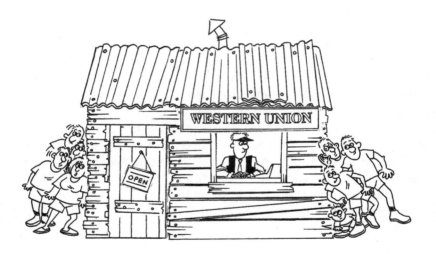

...and then jumping for joy when they hear you've finished it **all**?!

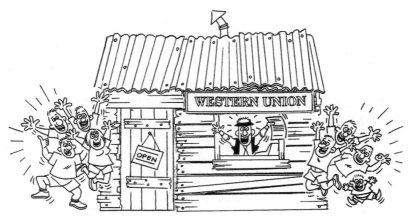

Because that's the only benefit they're ever going to get from you "cleaning your plate!"

Forget it! Nobody anywhere cares how much you're eating, and "cleaning your plate" won't do any of them the slightest bit of good!

"Then why do parents—especially Mommies—keep pushing it?"

Because, as we said earlier: some Mommies think their "precious" is always about 20 or 30 seconds away from total starvation anyway, and the only way they can prevent that is by getting you eating. And if it takes laying a "guilt trip" on you to make that happen—

"If the kid in Ethiopia got hold of that much food, **he'd** sure as heck finish it all, so why shouldn't **you**?!"

—then that's exactly what she'll do!

"Amazing!"

And what's the upshot of all this Einsteinian logic? Of course: you keep getting bigger and bigger and the kid in Ethiopia starves to death anyway. So show me the winner!

"OK. But aren't you forgetting one thing?"

What's that?

"—I paid good money for that food."

So?

"So, shouldn't I get my money's-**worth**?!"

Sure you should—

"I knew I'd 'get' you!"

—from everything else!

"Excuse me?"

Look, there's nothing wrong with getting your money's-worth from things that **enrich** your life—your house, your car, your computer, your camcorder, your dog.

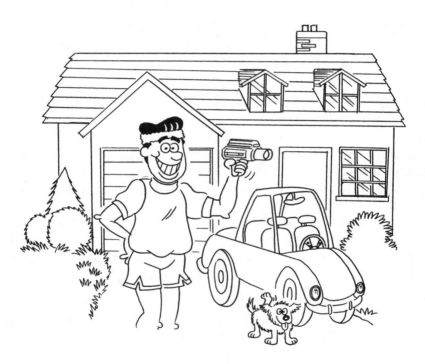

But overeating doesn't enrich your life, it **destroys** it!

So the more you try getting your money's-worth out of **food**, the more you **destroy** yourself! Which will **not** win you next year's Nobel Prize in Cleverness!

So stop doing it! Stop trying to get your money's-worth out of food, stop worrying about "wasting" it, stop claiming there's some "virtue" in cleaning your plate, stop—

"All right! Enough! I'll do it!"

No you won't.

"What do you mean I won't?! I just told you I would!"

And I'm telling you you won't!

"Why won't I?"

Because you're "too far gone"—we all are. We've been so brainwashed into believing that "cleaning your plate" and "not wasting food" are the most wonderful things we can do that we're helpless to **stop** doing them!

"Oooh—that's bad!"

No: that's good!

"That's 'good?!'"

Of course:

The fact is, you can't get where you're going till you know where you're at. And now that we **know** where you're at—that you're always going to be "cleaning your plate," no matter what—getting where you're going becomes easy:

Just put a minimum amount of food on that plate!

If that's not enough to satisfy you, you can always go back for a minimally-loaded second plate. Then a third. Then a fourth. And so on.

By starting out with a **minimum** amount of food, you at least give yourself a **chance** to be satisfied with less; a **chance** to avoid packing in unnecessary calories.

The other way—loading your plate to the "max"—it won't matter if you do get full halfway through: you're going to finish that mountain of mush come Hell or high water!

Why?

Because it's the "right thing to do!"

OK, fine; do it!

All we're saying is: Just finish a teensy-weensy plateful, instead of half the food in Fontana! If that's not enough to satisfy you, have another teensy-weensy plateful, then another. Like Jay Leno used to tell us, in those Doritos commericals: "Don't worry: we'll make more!"

And another thing:

If you're like most "devoted" eaters, the nerve endings in your stomach that are supposed to signal "fullness" to your brain have been so battered and beaten by your eating that they no longer do their job very well. As a result, you could be getting physically full after the first **third** of your "food mountain," and yet have **no way of knowing it** till you're almost finished, by which time it's too late.

So, in addition to doing what we've already suggested—taking your original "mountain" and dividing it up into, say, three or four little "hills"—we would ask you to do one more thing: take a reasonable **break** between each of those "hills."

Why?

To give your battered nerves the extra time they need, to do what they were originally designed to do.

Again, if you're still hungry, there's always more food to be had. But at least give yourself the **chance** to be satisfied with less.

At first, of course, you'll resent the fact that this new way of portioning out food is keeping you from eating the way you always have. I mean, food is your "love," your "buddy," and who likes to lose a "buddy?"

Well, all we can say is: if that one minimum plate of food is all your body needs, then let that be "buddy" enough! Push anything **more** on that body and you enter into the realm of, "With friends like that....!"

Our job is to get you fit and help you lose a little bodysize. A lifetime program of exercise walking will do just that, regardless of what you eat (within obvious limits). So don't for a minute think that we're **demanding** that you change the way you eat.

We offer the above only because it reveals something about most of us—an inability to "waste food," etc.—that, once known, can be easily dealt with—**if one chooses**!

And if you **don't** "choose"?

No problem: just keep walking!

2) The second way to avoid overeating is the easiest: just

Stay away from "all-you-can-eat" restaurants.

Since you always want to get your money's-worth out of everything, and since all-you-can-eat places are nothing more than "bottomless pits," you'll never feel you've gotten your money's-worth on less than 10 or 20 pounds of food!

Again: that attitude is never going to change, so avoid all-you-can-eat places like the Plague!

3) Another simple trick for changing your eating habits is to just delay your first feeding of the day for as long as you can.

Remember: the cravings you have for certain amounts or certain types of food are merely a creation of your Subconscious Mind to get you doing the same things day after day; they rarely have anything to do with a **real** need for food, your **body's** need for food, even though it feels like they do.

So what?

So, you won't be killing yourself if you ignore some of those cravings every now and then.

And what will that do?

Well, in the same way you "train" your Subconscious to make you **hungry** for an omelet at 7:30 tomorrow by having one at 7:30 today, so you can "train" your Subconscious to **not** make you hungry for an omelet at 7:30 tomorrow by **ignoring** the hunger you have for one at 7:30 today (which came about, most likely, because you had one at 7:30 yesterday!)

Your Subconscious will, of course, try again at 8 o'clock, then 8:30, then 9 o'clock, etc., because it thinks you really do need that omelet, to survive, and it wouldn't be doing its job if it didn't keep making you hungry for it.

And eventually, of course, you **will** give in to its demands because eventually you'll **have** to, to keep your energy up—which is the only reason food exists.

All we're saying is: try to give in to your Subconscious Mind's demands as **late** as possible, not as **early**, because virtually all of its demands will be false ones, and every false demand you can ignore on Day One will be one fewer false demand you'll have to deal with on Day Two.

Why?

Because every false demand you live through will show your Subconscious that you **don't** need to eat every half hour to get from one day to the next (normal eaters certainly don't!), and it will stop trying to make you do so.

In other words, you will make "not eating" as much of a habit as "eating" ever was, and any time you can make something a habit, so that doing it becomes automatic, your race is all but won.

Look, it's really simple:

> **The more you eat, the more you**
> **want to eat,**
> **need to eat,**
> **can eat;**

> **The less you eat, the less you**
> **want to eat,**
> **need to eat,**
> **can eat.**

These are Laws of Nature; they can't be broken:

You get along on less by "training" your body to get along on less—not by stuffing yourself! The more you have today, the **more** you'll want tomorrow; the less you have today, the **less** you'll want tomorrow.

As we've said, your Subconscious Mind takes notes on what you eat each day. If you survive to the next day, it assumes you did so **because** of what you ate. So, to get you to tomorrow, all it has to do is get you eating those same things all over again, thinking that's what you need to eat, to survive.

That pattern is never going to change. You can use this knowledge to your advantage and start ignoring some of these false demands,

OR

You can keep giving in to them, believing you're "really hungry" for hotcakes-and-bacon at 7:30, a couple of donuts at 9, a fudge brownie at 10, a double cheeseburger-and-fries at 11:30, a tuna sandwich at 2, a bag of peanuts at 3, a candy bar at 4, etc., and that, if you didn't satisfy these "real hungers," you'd starve to death!

Either way, it makes no difference to us.

Our job here is to get you fit and, if possible, help you lose a little bodysize, and that you can do without ever skipping a meal. All you **have** to do is go out for a Fitwalk every day and you can kiss that bodysize good-bye forever!

It's just that, if you **can** change your eating habits a little bit, you can kiss it good-bye that much **sooner**.

And isn't there someone you know who'd get a kick out of **that**?!

30

"No Sweat!"

There's a craze that rears its silly-but-dangerous head from time to time and that you should be on the lookout for: people trying to convince you that you can **sweat** your bodysize off!

Those pushing this insanity count on you knowing two things:

1) people who exercise **sweat**, and
2) people who exercise **lose bodysize**.

What they then try to make you believe is that it's the **sweating** that's leading to the bodysize loss, not the **exercise**!

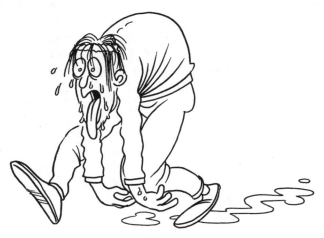

So, their next step becomes simple: just sell you something—most often, an airtight suit—that will get you sweating like Niagara the minute you so much as **think** about moving a muscle!

No problem there, except: by doing **one** thing—artificially increasing the amount you sweat—they're actually **keeping** you from doing the other: losing weight!

"What?"

Absolutely:

The only "weight" worth losing is "fat"—or, as we term it, "bodysize." Whatever weight you lose in the form of "water"—a.k.a., "sweat"—had better be replaced right after you've lost it, or the only exercise you'll soon be doing deals strictly with daisies!

The only way you lose bodysize is by burning calories: the more calories you burn, the more bodysize you lose; the fewer you burn, the less you lose. Laws of Nature.

So, anything that **keeps** you from burning calories actually **keeps** you from losing bodysize.

And what would **keep** you from burning calories?

Well, why do we burn calories in the first place?"

1) To maintain an internal temperature of 98.6°F. (37°C.)

Obviously, anything that **helps** your body maintain that temperature—by holding heat in with airtight clothing, for example—relieves your body of the need to burn **calories** to do so.

Thus, the more heat you hold in, the fewer calories your **body** has to burn to keep you warm, and the less bodysize you lose.

2) To provide energy for your muscles.

Muscles are designed to work best—and burn the most calories—at some optimum temperature (that same 98.6°F.). Raise that temperature, by holding in heat, and those muscles **won't** be working at their max.

And how do you raise that temperature? Of course: by holding heat **in** instead of letting it escape.

Again: the **more** heat you hold in, the more heat accumulates around the muscles, and the **fewer** calories they can burn, which means the **less** fat you lose.

"So, what am I supposed to do: go running around naked when it's 20 below?!"

No: we're shooting for **fit** people here, not **dead** ones!

All you have to do, to be in the proper "sweat zone," is wear just enough clothing to be "comfortable" at the start of your walk—not too hot, not too cold. As long as you're "comfortable" at the start, then the amount you sweat will be the "right" amount, the "natural" amount.

In other words: all your sweat will be due to "calories burned" ("good sweat") and not "heat unable to escape" ("bad sweat.") And the **amount** you sweat will be an accurate indication of how much bodysize you're **losing**—rather than how much bodysize you're **keeping** yourself from losing!

So always dress in a way where you expose as much of your skin as possible to the air, but not at the risk of freezing to death!

Do that, and you'll do just fine!

31

If You Smoke

If you smoke, you shouldn't.

Of course, if you've figured out which end of the cigarette to light, you already know that.

However, if you not only smoke but are plus-sized on top of it, then you're **really** tempting fate, and you might want to do **something** about reducing that "double jeopardy!"

Since smoking is such a hard habit to kick—harder than heroin, according to those who know—let's forget about that one for a moment and work on the other one: your size.

Like your non-smoking neighbors, the solution to that problem is easy: exercise.

Which exercise?

Well, what would you say about an exercise that not only helped you lose bodysize in the shortest time possible, but would **let you smoke while you were doing it** (save your breath: as a former smoker, we already know the answer!)?

Naturally, you probably won't be able to walk as fast or as far as someone your size and age who doesn't smoke. That's OK: you're only walking to get fit and lose a little bodysize, not set the land speed record, so who cares how long it takes to happen, as long as it happens without you having to give up one of your favorite pastimes?

So go out there and enjoy those cigarettes—every Fitwalking step of the way!

If, some day, you can give up smoking, all the better. But if you can't, no problem: just keep walking!

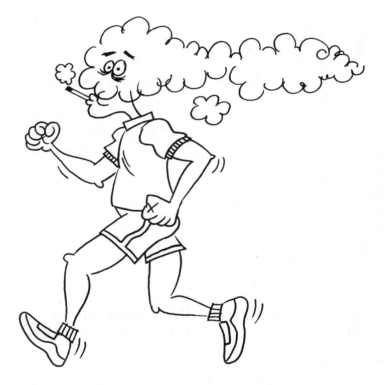

32

"It's a Boy!"

One of life's great joys can be: having children.

And it can be even **more** joyous if you can stay as trim as possible the whole nine months.

There are obviously two ways to control your figure during pregnancy: eating less or exercising more.

If anyone reading this thinks that eating less during pregnancy is a smashing idea, would you please leave your name with the corrections officer on your way out? Thanks.

I guess if you're a board-certified nutritionist, you can point to your food and state with certainty that "This can go" but "This must stay."

Me? I say: why take a chance? Why not give the little guy inside you all the good food you can, and then let **him** "tell" you what he needs or doesn't need?

Which only leaves "exercising more," if you want to stay as trim as possible during pregnancy, and return to trimness as soon as possible thereafter.

We already know that, in the long run, Fitwalking wins out over every other exercise. But it can be just as big a winner in the short run—specifically, the short run known as "pregnancy."

The reason for this is that you'd like to be doing an exercise almost to the time of delivery, without feeling like you're "delivering" every time you do the exercise (those of you who've tried aerobic dancing in your eighth month know exactly what I'm talking about!)

If there was ever a less jarring way than Fitwalking to maintain body size without harming the baby, I'm not aware of it. In fact, I sometimes think that Fitwalking is God's gift to pregnant women, and that all the rest of us are just borrowing it for a little while!

And its value is more than just "cosmetic:"

It's a known fact that, all else being equal, **fit** women have an easier time, delivering, than **non**-fit women. So, not only does Fitwalking help keep you looking good without hurting the baby, it also makes it easier to bring that baby into the world.

So if you want to stay as trim as possible during pregnancy, without depriving your baby of any nutrients; want to help your delivery; and want to get back into shape as quickly as possible after the baby is born, you have only one choice—and it's not: "pink" or "blue?"

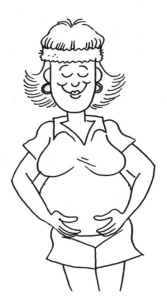

33

When You're Fit

With all other size-loss programs, it's: "**If** you lose bodysize..."

With Fitwalking, it's: "**When** you lose bodysize..."

Since your size loss is inevitable, you can start working out, ahead of time, what your new life will consist of.

The first thing you'll have to do is come up with a set of clever responses to all the compliments you'll be receiving.

A few that we like are:

"It went off the same way it went on: an ounce at a time. Nobody seemed to notice, while it was going on, but we're sure glad to hear how you feel, now that it's started coming off!"

"To be honest, I wish I had started sooner!"

"...and I **feel** a whole lot better, too!"

"I'd **love** to have lunch with you!"

—and so on.

The next thing you'll have to do is re-map your walking routes, to take in all the full-length windows you may have avoided when you were plus-sized.

113

That's OK: You won't admire yourself for more than five or ten minutes in each one, so there's almost no chance of your children starving to death before you get back, unless, of course, you haven't fed them yet this month.

Should you feel guilty, spending so much time admiring yourself? Not at all! Why else did you lose all that bodysize?!

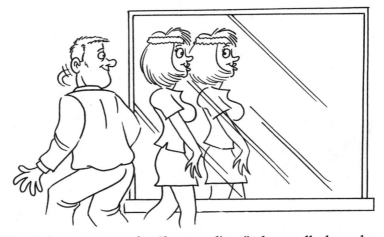

Which brings us to the "bottom line:" above all else, plan on **enjoying** your new life. I defy anyone to prove that we were put on this planet for any reason other than to enjoy it.

And, in a "private moment," be quietly grateful that you were lucky enough and courageous enough to have pulled yourself out of a hole that had no bottom; to have given yourself a life you can look forward to living each day; to have **walked yourself fit**!

34
A Final Word

So this is what the rest of your life will look like:

1) You will Fitwalk every day, going as fast as you comfortably can for as long as you comfortably can.

2) You will walk for any reason you want to, except one: to lose bodysize!

3) You will make no drastic changes in your eating habits, unless you feel you can do so without endangering your Fitwalking.

4) You will never weigh yourself.

5) You will lose one or two ounces of bodysize each day, until the inevitable day that you're down to a more manageable body size.

6) You will never see any change in your body—nor will you expect to—from the day you start your Fitwalking Program till the day you're down to the body size you'd like to be.

7) You will keep a record of your progress, if that suits you, but will never be a "slave" to it; never let it keep you on the couch, when you should be on the street, track, etc.

8) When you're ready, you'll try every other exercise you think you might enjoy—and might benefit from.

9) You will dress in a way that **minimizes** sweating, so you can **maximize** "calorie burn."

10) If you do decide to go on a "diet," sometime during your Fitwalking program, you will promise yourself that, if that less-than-effective "diet" makes you so discouraged that it threatens your guaranteed-effective Fitwalking, you will abandon that "diet" immediately and return to just walking yourself fit.

You will find that the beauty of Fitwalking—and the thing that makes it so different from all other size-loss programs—especially "diets"—is that it **builds on itself**:

The more you do, the more you **can** do;

The more bodysize you lose, the more bodysize you **can** lose and **do** lose.

And only one thing is required: that you begin!

And once you do begin, we see no reason why you won't quickly join the ranks of other Fitwalkers, who've made the greatest discovery of all about Fitwalking:

The more you do it, the more you **want** to do it.

—a little bit like—well, that's a subject for another book!

For now, just get out and

Walk Yourself Fit!

—and make your whole **World** a happier place to live!

35

The Log

What follows is a Weekly Log for charting your Fitwalking progress.

We've made it as easy as possible for you to "keep" this log; for example, lots of check marks instead of essay questions. We would, however, ask you to be as complete as you can in the sections requiring your comments.

If you don't want to write in this book—if, for example, you don't own it—just photocopy a two-page "set" of Log pages as many times as you need to and create your own Log book.

As you'll notice, our main concern is with "subjective" impressions ("you" being the "subject"): how you feel, overall; how your legs feel; how easy your walk was; etc.
Though we've also allocated space for "objective" results—things evaluated by some "object" (like a "stopwatch" or a "yardstick")—we consider those far less important than finding out how **you** are changing from week to week (which is why most of these "objective" measurements are placed at the bottom of the page and are labeled "Optional.")

Anyway, have fun with the Log and enjoy what it's telling you as you Walk Yourself Fit!

Week No.:_____   Date: _____   Approx. Time of Day: _____ to _____

About how far did you walk today?_____

How does that distance compare with how far you walked a week ago?
❏ Much farther   ❏ About the same
❏ A little farther   ❏ Not as far

About how fast did you walk today (on average?)
❏ Over 30 min./mile   ❏ 20-25 min./mile   ❏ 15-16 min./mile   ❏ 10-12 min./mile
❏ 25-30 min./mile   ❏ 17-19 min./mile   ❏ 13-14 min./mile   ❏ Less than 10

How does this compare with how fast you walked a week ago?
❏ Much faster   ❏ About the same
❏ A little faster   ❏ A little slower

How did your leg muscles feel at the start of your walk?
❏ Loose and "fluid"   ❏ Somewhat "stiff"   ❏ Painful
❏ About "normal"   ❏ Very "stiff"   ❏ "Tired" or "Empty"

How did your leg muscles feel at the mid-point of your walk?
❏ Loose and "fluid"   ❏ Somewhat "stiff"   ❏ Painful
❏ About "normal"   ❏ Very "stiff"   ❏ "Tired" or "Empty"

How did your leg muscles feel at the end of your walk?
❏ Loose and "fluid"   ❏ Somewhat "stiff"   ❏ Painful
❏ About "normal"   ❏ Very "stiff"   ❏ "Tired" or "Empty"

How would you describe the way you were breathing at the "height" of your walk?
❏ With great difficulty   ❏ "Normally"
❏ With some difficulty   ❏ Very easily

What clothing size were you able to fit into this morning?
❏ Slack size:
❏ Dress size (if applicable):

How would you describe the "fit?"
❏ Very tight   ❏ "Just right"   ❏ Very loose
❏ Somewhat tight   ❏ A bit loose   ❏ Walked right out of them!

Overall Impressions and Comments on Your Progress:

Optional Walking Log: Lap Length: _____

Lap No.	1	2	3	4	5	6	7	8
Lap Time								
Cum. Time								

Comments:

Week No.:_____   Date: _____   Approx. Time of Day: _____ to _____

About how far did you walk today?_____

How does that distance compare with how far you walked a week ago?
      ❏ Much farther   ❏ About the same
      ❏ A little farther   ❏ Not as far

About how fast did you walk today (on average?)
❏ Over 30 min./mile   ❏ 20-25 min./mile   ❏ 15-16 min./mile   ❏ 10-12 min./mile
❏ 25-30 min./mile   ❏ 17-19 min./mile   ❏ 13-14 min./mile   ❏ Less than 10

How does this compare with how fast you walked a week ago?
      ❏ Much faster   ❏ About the same
      ❏ A little faster   ❏ A little slower

How did your leg muscles feel at the start of your walk?
      ❏ Loose and "fluid"   ❏ Somewhat "stiff"   ❏ Painful
      ❏ About "normal"   ❏ Very "stiff"   ❏ "Tired" or "Empty"

How did your leg muscles feel at the mid-point of your walk?
      ❏ Loose and "fluid"   ❏ Somewhat "stiff"   ❏ Painful
      ❏ About "normal"   ❏ Very "stiff"   ❏ "Tired" or "Empty"

How did your leg muscles feel at the end of your walk?
      ❏ Loose and "fluid"   ❏ Somewhat "stiff"   ❏ Painful
      ❏ About "normal"   ❏ Very "stiff"   ❏ "Tired" or "Empty"

How would you describe the way you were breathing at the "height" of your walk?
      ❏ With great difficulty   ❏ "Normally"
      ❏ With some difficulty   ❏ Very easily

What clothing size were you able to fit into this morning?
      ❏ Slack size:
      ❏ Dress size (if applicable):

How would you describe the "fit?"
      ❏ Very tight   ❏ "Just right"   ❏ Very loose
      ❏ Somewhat tight   ❏ A bit loose   ❏ Walked right out of them!

Overall Impressions and Comments on Your Progress:

Optional Walking Log: Lap Length: _____

Lap No.	1	2	3	4	5	6	7	8
Lap Time								
Cum. Time								

Comments:

Week No.:_____   Date: _____   Approx. Time of Day: _____ to _____

About how far did you walk today?_____

How does that distance compare with how far you walked a week ago?
- ❏ Much farther
- ❏ A little farther
- ❏ About the same
- ❏ Not as far

About how fast did you walk today (on average?)
- ❏ Over 30 min./mile
- ❏ 25-30 min./mile
- ❏ 20-25 min./mile
- ❏ 17-19 min./mile
- ❏ 15-16 min./mile
- ❏ 13-14 min./mile
- ❏ 10-12 min./mile
- ❏ Less than 10

How does this compare with how fast you walked a week ago?
- ❏ Much faster
- ❏ A little faster
- ❏ About the same
- ❏ A little slower

How did your leg muscles feel at the start of your walk?
- ❏ Loose and "fluid"
- ❏ About "normal"
- ❏ Somewhat "stiff"
- ❏ Very "stiff"
- ❏ Painful
- ❏ "Tired" or "Empty"

How did your leg muscles feel at the mid-point of your walk?
- ❏ Loose and "fluid"
- ❏ About "normal"
- ❏ Somewhat "stiff"
- ❏ Very "stiff"
- ❏ Painful
- ❏ "Tired" or "Empty"

How did your leg muscles feel at the end of your walk?
- ❏ Loose and "fluid"
- ❏ About "normal"
- ❏ Somewhat "stiff"
- ❏ Very "stiff"
- ❏ Painful
- ❏ "Tired" or "Empty"

How would you describe the way you were breathing at the "height" of your walk?
- ❏ With great difficulty
- ❏ With some difficulty
- ❏ "Normally"
- ❏ Very easily

What clothing size were you able to fit into this morning?
- ❏ Slack size:
- ❏ Dress size (if applicable):

How would you describe the "fit?"
- ❏ Very tight
- ❏ Somewhat tight
- ❏ "Just right"
- ❏ A bit loose
- ❏ Very loose
- ❏ Walked right out of them!

Overall Impressions and Comments on Your Progress:

Optional Walking Log: Lap Length: _____

Lap No.	1	2	3	4	5	6	7	8
Lap Time								
Cum. Time								

Comments:

Week No.:_____   Date: _____   Approx. Time of Day: _____ to _____

About how far did you walk today?_____

How does that distance compare with how far you walked a week ago?
- ❏ Much farther   ❏ About the same
- ❏ A little farther   ❏ Not as far

About how fast did you walk today (on average?)
- ❏ Over 30 min./mile   ❏ 20-25 min./mile   ❏ 15-16 min./mile   ❏ 10-12 min./mile
- ❏ 25-30 min./mile   ❏ 17-19 min./mile   ❏ 13-14 min./mile   ❏ Less than 10

How does this compare with how fast you walked a week ago?
- ❏ Much faster   ❏ About the same
- ❏ A little faster   ❏ A little slower

How did your leg muscles feel at the start of your walk?
- ❏ Loose and "fluid"   ❏ Somewhat "stiff"   ❏ Painful
- ❏ About "normal"   ❏ Very "stiff"   ❏ "Tired" or "Empty"

How did your leg muscles feel at the mid-point of your walk?
- ❏ Loose and "fluid"   ❏ Somewhat "stiff"   ❏ Painful
- ❏ About "normal"   ❏ Very "stiff"   ❏ "Tired" or "Empty"

How did your leg muscles feel at the end of your walk?
- ❏ Loose and "fluid"   ❏ Somewhat "stiff"   ❏ Painful
- ❏ About "normal"   ❏ Very "stiff"   ❏ "Tired" or "Empty"

How would you describe the way you were breathing at the "height" of your walk?
- ❏ With great difficulty   ❏ "Normally"
- ❏ With some difficulty   ❏ Very easily

What clothing size were you able to fit into this morning?
- ❏ Slack size:
- ❏ Dress size (if applicable):

How would you describe the "fit?"
- ❏ Very tight   ❏ "Just right"   ❏ Very loose
- ❏ Somewhat tight   ❏ A bit loose   ❏ Walked right out of them!

Overall Impressions and Comments on Your Progress:

Optional Walking Log: Lap Length: _____

Lap No.	1	2	3	4	5	6	7	8
Lap Time								
Cum. Time								

Comments:

Week No.:_____ Date: _____ Approx. Time of Day: _____ to _____

About how far did you walk today?_____

How does that distance compare with how far you walked a week ago?
❑ Much farther   ❑ About the same
❑ A little farther   ❑ Not as far

About how fast did you walk today (on average?)
❑ Over 30 min./mile   ❑ 20-25 min./mile   ❑ 15-16 min./mile   ❑ 10-12 min./mile
❑ 25-30 min./mile   ❑ 17-19 min./mile   ❑ 13-14 min./mile   ❑ Less than 10

How does this compare with how fast you walked a week ago?
❑ Much faster   ❑ About the same
❑ A little faster   ❑ A little slower

How did your leg muscles feel at the start of your walk?
❑ Loose and "fluid"   ❑ Somewhat "stiff"   ❑ Painful
❑ About "normal"   ❑ Very "stiff"   ❑ "Tired" or "Empty"

How did your leg muscles feel at the mid-point of your walk?
❑ Loose and "fluid"   ❑ Somewhat "stiff"   ❑ Painful
❑ About "normal"   ❑ Very "stiff"   ❑ "Tired" or "Empty"

How did your leg muscles feel at the end of your walk?
❑ Loose and "fluid"   ❑ Somewhat "stiff"   ❑ Painful
❑ About "normal"   ❑ Very "stiff"   ❑ "Tired" or "Empty"

How would you describe the way you were breathing at the "height" of your walk?
❑ With great difficulty   ❑ "Normally"
❑ With some difficulty   ❑ Very easily

What clothing size were you able to fit into this morning?
❑ Slack size:
❑ Dress size (if applicable):

How would you describe the "fit?"
❑ Very tight   ❑ "Just right"   ❑ Very loose
❑ Somewhat tight   ❑ A bit loose   ❑ Walked right out of them!

Overall Impressions and Comments on Your Progress:

Optional Walking Log: Lap Length: _____

Lap No.	1	2	3	4	5	6	7	8
Lap Time								
Cum. Time								

Comments:

Week No.:_____   Date: _____   Approx. Time of Day: _____ to _____

About how far did you walk today?_____

How does that distance compare with how far you walked a week ago?
❏ Much farther   ❏ About the same
❏ A little farther   ❏ Not as far

About how fast did you walk today (on average?)
❏ Over 30 min./mile   ❏ 20-25 min./mile   ❏ 15-16 min./mile   ❏ 10-12 min./mile
❏ 25-30 min./mile   ❏ 17-19 min./mile   ❏ 13-14 min./mile   ❏ Less than 10

How does this compare with how fast you walked a week ago?
❏ Much faster   ❏ About the same
❏ A little faster   ❏ A little slower

How did your leg muscles feel at the start of your walk?
❏ Loose and "fluid"   ❏ Somewhat "stiff"   ❏ Painful
❏ About "normal"   ❏ Very "stiff"   ❏ "Tired" or "Empty"

How did your leg muscles feel at the mid-point of your walk?
❏ Loose and "fluid"   ❏ Somewhat "stiff"   ❏ Painful
❏ About "normal"   ❏ Very "stiff"   ❏ "Tired" or "Empty"

How did your leg muscles feel at the end of your walk?
❏ Loose and "fluid"   ❏ Somewhat "stiff"   ❏ Painful
❏ About "normal"   ❏ Very "stiff"   ❏ "Tired" or "Empty"

How would you describe the way you were breathing at the "height" of your walk?
❏ With great difficulty   ❏ "Normally"
❏ With some difficulty   ❏ Very easily

What clothing size were you able to fit into this morning?
❏ Slack size:
❏ Dress size (if applicable):

How would you describe the "fit?"
❏ Very tight   ❏ "Just right"   ❏ Very loose
❏ Somewhat tight   ❏ A bit loose   ❏ Walked right out of them!

Overall Impressions and Comments on Your Progress:

Optional Walking Log: Lap Length: _____

Lap No.	1	2	3	4	5	6	7	8
Lap Time								
Cum. Time								

Comments:

Week No.:_____   Date: _____   Approx. Time of Day: _____ to _____

About how far did you walk today?_____

How does that distance compare with how far you walked a week ago?
❏ Much farther   ❏ About the same
❏ A little farther   ❏ Not as far

About how fast did you walk today (on average?)
❏ Over 30 min./mile   ❏ 20-25 min./mile   ❏ 15-16 min./mile   ❏ 10-12 min./mile
❏ 25-30 min./mile   ❏ 17-19 min./mile   ❏ 13-14 min./mile   ❏ Less than 10

How does this compare with how fast you walked a week ago?
❏ Much faster   ❏ About the same
❏ A little faster   ❏ A little slower

How did your leg muscles feel at the start of your walk?
❏ Loose and "fluid"   ❏ Somewhat "stiff"   ❏ Painful
❏ About "normal"   ❏ Very "stiff"   ❏ "Tired" or "Empty"

How did your leg muscles feel at the mid-point of your walk?
❏ Loose and "fluid"   ❏ Somewhat "stiff"   ❏ Painful
❏ About "normal"   ❏ Very "stiff"   ❏ "Tired" or "Empty"

How did your leg muscles feel at the end of your walk?
❏ Loose and "fluid"   ❏ Somewhat "stiff"   ❏ Painful
❏ About "normal"   ❏ Very "stiff"   ❏ "Tired" or "Empty"

How would you describe the way you were breathing at the "height" of your walk?
❏ With great difficulty   ❏ "Normally"
❏ With some difficulty   ❏ Very easily

What clothing size were you able to fit into this morning?
❏ Slack size:
❏ Dress size (if applicable):

How would you describe the "fit?"
❏ Very tight   ❏ "Just right"   ❏ Very loose
❏ Somewhat tight   ❏ A bit loose   ❏ Walked right out of them!

Overall Impressions and Comments on Your Progress:

Optional Walking Log: Lap Length: _____

Lap No.	1	2	3	4	5	6	7	8
Lap Time								
Cum. Time								

Comments:

Week No.:_____   Date: _____   Approx. Time of Day: _____ to _____

About how far did you walk today?_____

How does that distance compare with how far you walked a week ago?
    ❏ Much farther   ❏ About the same
    ❏ A little farther   ❏ Not as far

About how fast did you walk today (on average?)
❏ Over 30 min./mile ❏ 20-25 min./mile ❏ 15-16 min./mile ❏ 10-12 min./mile
❏ 25-30 min./mile ❏ 17-19 min./mile ❏ 13-14 min./mile ❏ Less than 10

How does this compare with how fast you walked a week ago?
    ❏ Much faster   ❏ About the same
    ❏ A little faster   ❏ A little slower

How did your leg muscles feel at the start of your walk?
   ❏ Loose and "fluid" ❏ Somewhat "stiff" ❏ Painful
   ❏ About "normal"   ❏ Very "stiff"   ❏ "Tired" or "Empty"

How did your leg muscles feel at the mid-point of your walk?
   ❏ Loose and "fluid" ❏ Somewhat "stiff" ❏ Painful
   ❏ About "normal"   ❏ Very "stiff"   ❏ "Tired" or "Empty"

How did your leg muscles feel at the end of your walk?
   ❏ Loose and "fluid" ❏ Somewhat "stiff" ❏ Painful
   ❏ About "normal"   ❏ Very "stiff"   ❏ "Tired" or "Empty"

How would you describe the way you were breathing at the "height" of your walk?
    ❏ With great difficulty   ❏ "Normally"
    ❏ With some difficulty   ❏ Very easily

What clothing size were you able to fit into this morning?
    ❏ Slack size:
    ❏ Dress size (if applicable):

How would you describe the "fit?"
   ❏ Very tight   ❏ "Just right"   ❏ Very loose
   ❏ Somewhat tight   ❏ A bit loose   ❏ Walked right out of them!

Overall Impressions and Comments on Your Progress:

Optional Walking Log: Lap Length: _____

Lap No.	1	2	3	4	5	6	7	8
Lap Time								
Cum. Time								

Comments:

Week No.:_____   Date: _____   Approx. Time of Day: _____ to _____

About how far did you walk today?_____

How does that distance compare with how far you walked a week ago?
- ❏ Much farther   ❏ About the same
- ❏ A little farther   ❏ Not as far

About how fast did you walk today (on average?)
- ❏ Over 30 min./mile   ❏ 20-25 min./mile   ❏ 15-16 min./mile   ❏ 10-12 min./mile
- ❏ 25-30 min./mile   ❏ 17-19 min./mile   ❏ 13-14 min./mile   ❏ Less than 10

How does this compare with how fast you walked a week ago?
- ❏ Much faster   ❏ About the same
- ❏ A little faster   ❏ A little slower

How did your leg muscles feel at the start of your walk?
- ❏ Loose and "fluid"   ❏ Somewhat "stiff"   ❏ Painful
- ❏ About "normal"   ❏ Very "stiff"   ❏ "Tired" or "Empty"

How did your leg muscles feel at the mid-point of your walk?
- ❏ Loose and "fluid"   ❏ Somewhat "stiff"   ❏ Painful
- ❏ About "normal"   ❏ Very "stiff"   ❏ "Tired" or "Empty"

How did your leg muscles feel at the end of your walk?
- ❏ Loose and "fluid"   ❏ Somewhat "stiff"   ❏ Painful
- ❏ About "normal"   ❏ Very "stiff"   ❏ "Tired" or "Empty"

How would you describe the way you were breathing at the "height" of your walk?
- ❏ With great difficulty   ❏ "Normally"
- ❏ With some difficulty   ❏ Very easily

What clothing size were you able to fit into this morning?
- ❏ Slack size:
- ❏ Dress size (if applicable):

How would you describe the "fit?"
- ❏ Very tight   ❏ "Just right"   ❏ Very loose
- ❏ Somewhat tight   ❏ A bit loose   ❏ Walked right out of them!

Overall Impressions and Comments on Your Progress:

Optional Walking Log: Lap Length: _____

Lap No.	1	2	3	4	5	6	7	8
Lap Time								
Cum. Time								

Comments:

Week No.:_____ Date: _____ Approx. Time of Day: _____ to _____

About how far did you walk today?_____

How does that distance compare with how far you walked a week ago?
    ❏ Much farther   ❏ About the same
    ❏ A little farther   ❏ Not as far

About how fast did you walk today (on average?)
❏ Over 30 min./mile   ❏ 20-25 min./mile   ❏ 15-16 min./mile   ❏ 10-12 min./mile
❏ 25-30 min./mile   ❏ 17-19 min./mile   ❏ 13-14 min./mile   ❏ Less than 10

How does this compare with how fast you walked a week ago?
    ❏ Much faster   ❏ About the same
    ❏ A little faster   ❏ A little slower

How did your leg muscles feel at the start of your walk?
    ❏ Loose and "fluid"   ❏ Somewhat "stiff"   ❏ Painful
    ❏ About "normal"   ❏ Very "stiff"   ❏ "Tired" or "Empty"

How did your leg muscles feel at the mid-point of your walk?
    ❏ Loose and "fluid"   ❏ Somewhat "stiff"   ❏ Painful
    ❏ About "normal"   ❏ Very "stiff"   ❏ "Tired" or "Empty"

How did your leg muscles feel at the end of your walk?
    ❏ Loose and "fluid"   ❏ Somewhat "stiff"   ❏ Painful
    ❏ About "normal"   ❏ Very "stiff"   ❏ "Tired" or "Empty"

How would you describe the way you were breathing at the "height" of your walk?
    ❏ With great difficulty   ❏ "Normally"
    ❏ With some difficulty   ❏ Very easily

What clothing size were you able to fit into this morning?
    ❏ Slack size:
    ❏ Dress size (if applicable):

How would you describe the "fit?"
    ❏ Very tight   ❏ "Just right"   ❏ Very loose
    ❏ Somewhat tight   ❏ A bit loose   ❏ Walked right out of them!

Overall Impressions and Comments on Your Progress:

Optional Walking Log: Lap Length: _____

Lap No.	1	2	3	4	5	6	7	8
Lap Time								
Cum. Time								

Comments:

Week No.:_____   Date: _____   Approx. Time of Day: _____ to _____

About how far did you walk today?_____

How does that distance compare with how far you walked a week ago?
❏ Much farther   ❏ About the same
❏ A little farther   ❏ Not as far

About how fast did you walk today (on average?)
❏ Over 30 min./mile   ❏ 20-25 min./mile   ❏ 15-16 min./mile   ❏ 10-12 min./mile
❏ 25-30 min./mile   ❏ 17-19 min./mile   ❏ 13-14 min./mile   ❏ Less than 10

How does this compare with how fast you walked a week ago?
❏ Much faster   ❏ About the same
❏ A little faster   ❏ A little slower

How did your leg muscles feel at the start of your walk?
❏ Loose and "fluid"   ❏ Somewhat "stiff"   ❏ Painful
❏ About "normal"   ❏ Very "stiff"   ❏ "Tired" or "Empty"

How did your leg muscles feel at the mid-point of your walk?
❏ Loose and "fluid"   ❏ Somewhat "stiff"   ❏ Painful
❏ About "normal"   ❏ Very "stiff"   ❏ "Tired" or "Empty"

How did your leg muscles feel at the end of your walk?
❏ Loose and "fluid"   ❏ Somewhat "stiff"   ❏ Painful
❏ About "normal"   ❏ Very "stiff"   ❏ "Tired" or "Empty"

How would you describe the way you were breathing at the "height" of your walk?
❏ With great difficulty   ❏ "Normally"
❏ With some difficulty   ❏ Very easily

What clothing size were you able to fit into this morning?
❏ Slack size:
❏ Dress size (if applicable):

How would you describe the "fit?"
❏ Very tight   ❏ "Just right"   ❏ Very loose
❏ Somewhat tight   ❏ A bit loose   ❏ Walked right out of them!

Overall Impressions and Comments on Your Progress:

Optional Walking Log: Lap Length: _____

Lap No.	1	2	3	4	5	6	7	8
Lap Time								
Cum. Time								

Comments:

Week No.:_____ Date: _____ Approx. Time of Day: _____ to _____

About how far did you walk today?_____

How does that distance compare with how far you walked a week ago?
- ❏ Much farther
- ❏ A little farther
- ❏ About the same
- ❏ Not as far

About how fast did you walk today (on average?)
- ❏ Over 30 min./mile
- ❏ 20-25 min./mile
- ❏ 15-16 min./mile
- ❏ 10-12 min./mile
- ❏ 25-30 min./mile
- ❏ 17-19 min./mile
- ❏ 13-14 min./mile
- ❏ Less than 10

How does this compare with how fast you walked a week ago?
- ❏ Much faster
- ❏ A little faster
- ❏ About the same
- ❏ A little slower

How did your leg muscles feel at the start of your walk?
- ❏ Loose and "fluid"
- ❏ About "normal"
- ❏ Somewhat "stiff"
- ❏ Very "stiff"
- ❏ Painful
- ❏ "Tired" or "Empty"

How did your leg muscles feel at the mid-point of your walk?
- ❏ Loose and "fluid"
- ❏ About "normal"
- ❏ Somewhat "stiff"
- ❏ Very "stiff"
- ❏ Painful
- ❏ "Tired" or "Empty"

How did your leg muscles feel at the end of your walk?
- ❏ Loose and "fluid"
- ❏ About "normal"
- ❏ Somewhat "stiff"
- ❏ Very "stiff"
- ❏ Painful
- ❏ "Tired" or "Empty"

How would you describe the way you were breathing at the "height" of your walk?
- ❏ With great difficulty
- ❏ With some difficulty
- ❏ "Normally"
- ❏ Very easily

What clothing size were you able to fit into this morning?
- ❏ Slack size:
- ❏ Dress size (if applicable):

How would you describe the "fit?"
- ❏ Very tight
- ❏ Somewhat tight
- ❏ "Just right"
- ❏ A bit loose
- ❏ Very loose
- ❏ Walked right out of them!

Overall Impressions and Comments on Your Progress:

Optional Walking Log: Lap Length: _____

Lap No.	1	2	3	4	5	6	7	8
Lap Time								
Cum. Time								

Comments:

Week No.:_____   Date: _____   Approx. Time of Day: _____ to _____

About how far did you walk today?_____

How does that distance compare with how far you walked a week ago?
- ❏ Much farther
- ❏ A little farther
- ❏ About the same
- ❏ Not as far

About how fast did you walk today (on average?)
- ❏ Over 30 min./mile
- ❏ 25-30 min./mile
- ❏ 20-25 min./mile
- ❏ 17-19 min./mile
- ❏ 15-16 min./mile
- ❏ 13-14 min./mile
- ❏ 10-12 min./mile
- ❏ Less than 10

How does this compare with how fast you walked a week ago?
- ❏ Much faster
- ❏ A little faster
- ❏ About the same
- ❏ A little slower

How did your leg muscles feel at the start of your walk?
- ❏ Loose and "fluid"
- ❏ About "normal"
- ❏ Somewhat "stiff"
- ❏ Very "stiff"
- ❏ Painful
- ❏ "Tired" or "Empty"

How did your leg muscles feel at the mid-point of your walk?
- ❏ Loose and "fluid"
- ❏ About "normal"
- ❏ Somewhat "stiff"
- ❏ Very "stiff"
- ❏ Painful
- ❏ "Tired" or "Empty"

How did your leg muscles feel at the end of your walk?
- ❏ Loose and "fluid"
- ❏ About "normal"
- ❏ Somewhat "stiff"
- ❏ Very "stiff"
- ❏ Painful
- ❏ "Tired" or "Empty"

How would you describe the way you were breathing at the "height" of your walk?
- ❏ With great difficulty
- ❏ With some difficulty
- ❏ "Normally"
- ❏ Very easily

What clothing size were you able to fit into this morning?
- ❏ Slack size:
- ❏ Dress size (if applicable):

How would you describe the "fit?"
- ❏ Very tight
- ❏ Somewhat tight
- ❏ "Just right"
- ❏ A bit loose
- ❏ Very loose
- ❏ Walked right out of them!

Overall Impressions and Comments on Your Progress:

Optional Walking Log: Lap Length: _____

Lap No.	1	2	3	4	5	6	7	8
Lap Time								
Cum. Time								

Comments:

Week No.:_____   Date: _____   Approx. Time of Day: _____ to _____

About how far did you walk today?_____

How does that distance compare with how far you walked a week ago?
      ❏ Much farther   ❏ About the same
      ❏ A little farther   ❏ Not as far

About how fast did you walk today (on average?)
❏ Over 30 min./mile   ❏ 20-25 min./mile   ❏ 15-16 min./mile   ❏ 10-12 min./mile
❏ 25-30 min./mile   ❏ 17-19 min./mile   ❏ 13-14 min./mile   ❏ Less than 10

How does this compare with how fast you walked a week ago?
      ❏ Much faster   ❏ About the same
      ❏ A little faster   ❏ A little slower

How did your leg muscles feel at the start of your walk?
    ❏ Loose and "fluid"   ❏ Somewhat "stiff"   ❏ Painful
    ❏ About "normal"   ❏ Very "stiff"   ❏ "Tired" or "Empty"

How did your leg muscles feel at the mid-point of your walk?
    ❏ Loose and "fluid"   ❏ Somewhat "stiff"   ❏ Painful
    ❏ About "normal"   ❏ Very "stiff"   ❏ "Tired" or "Empty"

How did your leg muscles feel at the end of your walk?
    ❏ Loose and "fluid"   ❏ Somewhat "stiff"   ❏ Painful
    ❏ About "normal"   ❏ Very "stiff"   ❏ "Tired" or "Empty"

How would you describe the way you were breathing at the "height" of your walk?
     ❏ With great difficulty   ❏ "Normally"
     ❏ With some difficulty   ❏ Very easily

What clothing size were you able to fit into this morning?
     ❏ Slack size:
     ❏ Dress size (if applicable):

How would you describe the "fit?"
  ❏ Very tight   ❏ "Just right"   ❏ Very loose
  ❏ Somewhat tight   ❏ A bit loose   ❏ Walked right out of them!

Overall Impressions and Comments on Your Progress:

Optional Walking Log: Lap Length: _____

Lap No.	1	2	3	4	5	6	7	8
Lap Time								
Cum. Time								

Comments:

Week No.:_____ Date: _____ Approx. Time of Day: _____ to _____

About how far did you walk today?_____

How does that distance compare with how far you walked a week ago?
- ❏ Much farther   ❏ About the same
- ❏ A little farther   ❏ Not as far

About how fast did you walk today (on average?)
- ❏ Over 30 min./mile   ❏ 20-25 min./mile   ❏ 15-16 min./mile   ❏ 10-12 min./mile
- ❏ 25-30 min./mile   ❏ 17-19 min./mile   ❏ 13-14 min./mile   ❏ Less than 10

How does this compare with how fast you walked a week ago?
- ❏ Much faster   ❏ About the same
- ❏ A little faster   ❏ A little slower

How did your leg muscles feel at the start of your walk?
- ❏ Loose and "fluid"   ❏ Somewhat "stiff"   ❏ Painful
- ❏ About "normal"   ❏ Very "stiff"   ❏ "Tired" or "Empty"

How did your leg muscles feel at the mid-point of your walk?
- ❏ Loose and "fluid"   ❏ Somewhat "stiff"   ❏ Painful
- ❏ About "normal"   ❏ Very "stiff"   ❏ "Tired" or "Empty"

How did your leg muscles feel at the end of your walk?
- ❏ Loose and "fluid"   ❏ Somewhat "stiff"   ❏ Painful
- ❏ About "normal"   ❏ Very "stiff"   ❏ "Tired" or "Empty"

How would you describe the way you were breathing at the "height" of your walk?
- ❏ With great difficulty   ❏ "Normally"
- ❏ With some difficulty   ❏ Very easily

What clothing size were you able to fit into this morning?
- ❏ Slack size:
- ❏ Dress size (if applicable):

How would you describe the "fit?"
- ❏ Very tight   ❏ "Just right"   ❏ Very loose
- ❏ Somewhat tight   ❏ A bit loose   ❏ Walked right out of them!

Overall Impressions and Comments on Your Progress:

Optional Walking Log: Lap Length: _____

Lap No.	1	2	3	4	5	6	7	8
Lap Time								
Cum. Time								

Comments:

Week No.:_____   Date: _____   Approx. Time of Day: _____ to _____

About how far did you walk today?_____

How does that distance compare with how far you walked a week ago?
- ❏ Much farther
- ❏ A little farther
- ❏ About the same
- ❏ Not as far

About how fast did you walk today (on average?)
- ❏ Over 30 min./mile
- ❏ 25-30 min./mile
- ❏ 20-25 min./mile
- ❏ 17-19 min./mile
- ❏ 15-16 min./mile
- ❏ 13-14 min./mile
- ❏ 10-12 min./mile
- ❏ Less than 10

How does this compare with how fast you walked a week ago?
- ❏ Much faster
- ❏ A little faster
- ❏ About the same
- ❏ A little slower

How did your leg muscles feel at the start of your walk?
- ❏ Loose and "fluid"
- ❏ About "normal"
- ❏ Somewhat "stiff"
- ❏ Very "stiff"
- ❏ Painful
- ❏ "Tired" or "Empty"

How did your leg muscles feel at the mid-point of your walk?
- ❏ Loose and "fluid"
- ❏ About "normal"
- ❏ Somewhat "stiff"
- ❏ Very "stiff"
- ❏ Painful
- ❏ "Tired" or "Empty"

How did your leg muscles feel at the end of your walk?
- ❏ Loose and "fluid"
- ❏ About "normal"
- ❏ Somewhat "stiff"
- ❏ Very "stiff"
- ❏ Painful
- ❏ "Tired" or "Empty"

How would you describe the way you were breathing at the "height" of your walk?
- ❏ With great difficulty
- ❏ With some difficulty
- ❏ "Normally"
- ❏ Very easily

What clothing size were you able to fit into this morning?
- ❏ Slack size:
- ❏ Dress size (if applicable):

How would you describe the "fit?"
- ❏ Very tight
- ❏ Somewhat tight
- ❏ "Just right"
- ❏ A bit loose
- ❏ Very loose
- ❏ Walked right out of them!

Overall Impressions and Comments on Your Progress:

Optional Walking Log: Lap Length: _____

Lap No.	1	2	3	4	5	6	7	8
Lap Time								
Cum. Time								

Comments:

Glossary

"Actual" Pounds: What a weighing scale tells you (see, for comparison, **Size-Pounds**.)

Addictive: The property of a substance that makes you want to consume it when you're not, and makes it impossible to **stop** consuming it once you've started.

Adults: People able to exert some control over their own lives.

Aerobic Exercise: Exercise which uses the large muscles of the body long enough and hard enough that substantial quantities of oxygen (air) are required.   Typical aerobic exercises: brisk walking; long-distance running; cycling; swimming; aerobic dancing.

All-you-can-eat Restaurants: "Bottomless pits," where you feel obligated to eat 20 or 30 pounds of food because they let you.

Anaerobic Exercise: Exercise done in short bursts, so that great quantities of oxygen (air) are not required for muscles to do their work. Examples: weightlifting; sprint races; tennis.

Animal Starch: See **Glycogen**.

Anti-Survival: Anything that hurts your chances of seeing tomorrow (see: **Starvation Diet**).

Anxiety: Feeling of helplessness that arises when you lose control of your life situation.

Arbuckle, Fatty: Silent-film comedian.

Bad Sweat: Sweat that comes from holding in body heat artificially (with airtight plastic suits, excess clothing, pore-sealing skin creams, etc.) Actually **reduces** the amount of real weight ("fat") that exercise is trying to burn off (see also: **Good Sweat**).

Bathroom Scale: Instrument invented during the Spanish Inquisition to measure torture.

Bockar, Dr. Joyce: Author of *The Last Best Diet Book*, which revealed "not wasting food" and the value of "cleaning your plate" to be the nonsense they truly are.

Body: Your constant companion.

Body Fat: Nature's reminder that excess calories don't always vanish from the Universe just because they vanish from sight!

Body Size: The size of your body.

Bodysize: The part of your body that you lose on the Walk Yourself Fit Program (known as "weight" on "diet" programs); measured in "size-pounds."

Bodysize-reduction Program: Method of reducing bodysize by exercise, which may or may not result in loss of weight (see: **"Walk Yourself Fit Program"**).

Bolt, Usain: World champion sprinter from Jamaica.

Break-in Period: The first two weeks of Fitwalking, where the maximum number of muscle fibers are torn down, with new ones eventually built in their place; period of maximum soreness and muscle fatigue until new muscles get "on line."

Burn-out (Muscle): Premature muscle "shutdown," due to trying too much too soon.

Bushelful: A unit of measure equal to four pecks.

Ca-ca County: Less-than-ideal place to live (see, for comparison: **La-la Land**).

Calorie: A unit of heat-energy that fuels everything we do: thought; muscle function; food processing; maintenance of body temperature; etc.; when "number ingested" exceeds "number used," the excess is stored as body fat.

Chafing at the Bit: What horses start doing when they're anxious to run.

Challenge: To ask more out of something than it normally delivers.

Christmas morning: Traditionally, the most joyous morning of the year over much of the World.

Clothing Sizes: One of the ways Fitwalkers measure their progress.

Conservation Overdrive: The mechanism your body uses to conserve stored calories in the face of anything that threatens them (starvation; "diets;" etc.)

Control: Enforcing limits on your own or others' thoughts or actions.

Cosmetic: Referring to surface features only.

Couch: Piece of household furniture, designed for comfort.

Couch Potato: Someone who spends vast amounts of time on a certain piece of household furniture, watching people on TV who look the way he dreams of looking.

"Creature from the Black Lagoon:" Popular movie of the 1950's.

Cross-country Skiing: Terrific exercise that a lot of people talk about doing someday.

"Curiosity killed the Cat:" Time-honored expression suggesting that some things are better left alone.

Cutback: Reduction in the number of calories you normally eat (see also: **Hold-back**).

Daily Routine: Things you just do every day, without giving them a second thought (brushing your teeth; taking a shower; Fitwalking; etc.).

David: In the Bible: real short guy who specialized in killing real tall guys (see also: **Goliath**).

Des Moines: City in Iowa, supposedly typical of "middle America."

Diet: What you eat.

"Diet:" A program that **changes** what you eat, in an effort to help you lose weight.

Double Bonus (from walking yourself fit): 1) Easier to do than "dieting;" 2) A healthier You when you get there.

Double Jeopardy: Refers here to what a person places himself into when he not only is overweight, but smokes as well.

Double Overkill: When your body 1) restocks your muscles with more "power molecules" than your walk took out, and 2) builds stronger muscles than your walk tore down; the reason you can walk farther and faster on Day Fifty-one than you could on Day One.

Dream-world Slimming: Losing pounds-per-day, day after day; i.e., something that can only happen in your dreams (see, for contrast: **Real-world Slimming**).

Einstein, Albert: World-famous physicist who developed the Laws of Relativity.

Einstein's Corollary: "Everything is relative!" Applies to evaluating amount of bodysize an area has lost. Example: If lower chest has lost four inches, but waistline only one, waistline will actually appear to have gotten three inches **bigger** (see also: **Murphy's Law of Bodysize Loss**).

Endurance: Ability to continue a given activity for longer and longer periods of time.

Enemy: A non-friend: someone who is out to harm or hinder you. Refers here to what the Subconscious Mind seems to become when you try to "diet" your bodysize off.

Ethiopia: Nation in East Africa known for mass starvations due to combination of long-term drought and civil war; main reason why millions of young Americans are told to "clean their plate" at every meal.

Evolution: The horse we all rode in on.

Exercise: Method of losing bodysize by **using** calories rather than **restricting** them (see also: **"Diet."**)

Exercise Pushers: People who try to get you fit and losing bodysize by having you do something **positive**—"exercise"— rather than something **negative**: "starvation."

Expectations: Birthplace of disappointment.

False Hunger: Physical feeling, generated by your Subconscious Mind, to satisfy its mental needs (psychological "survival.")

Fargo: Pleasant town in North Dakota.

Fat: Chemical that evolution has chosen for us to use, to store most of our excess energy.

Fire Below: An intense longing in your gut for a particular substance (food; drug; etc.)

Fitness: Measure of your ability to meet life's challenges, both physical and mental.

Fitwalk: What you go on, to walk yourself fit.

Fitwalkers: People walking themselves fit.

Fitwalking: Walking as fast as you comfortably can for as long as you comfortably can.

Fitwalking Story: Exercised muscles pulling fat from storage to "recharge their batteries" and build themselves up.

Fontana: Town in Southern California.

Forbidden Fruit: Food whose consumption you can't honestly control and don't really want to.

Future: Something to look forward to or to dread, depending on what you do each day to shape it.

Gazelle: Fast-moving animal that bounds through forest and plain.

Glacier: The couch potato of rivers.

Glycogen: Also known as "animal starch;" stored in muscle and liver; made up of long strands of sugar molecules, strung together like beads in a necklace, which provide the quick energy needed for muscle movement, thought, etc.

Goal: The best way to bring order out of chaos.

Goliath: In the Bible: real tall guy who had a lot of trouble with real short guys (see also: **David**).

"Gonzo:" Anything done to excess.

Good Sweat: Sweat that results from "calories being burned", rather than "heat being trapped;" encouraged by wearing the minimum amount of clothing while exercising (see, for contrast: **Bad Sweat**).

Grapefruit-and-cottage cheese: Terrific way to lose weight permanently for a week or two.

Guaranteed Ounce: Amount of daily bodysize loss that Fitwalking can offer (see, for contrast: **Pipedream Pound**).

Habit: Anything you do automatically, day after day.

Heartbreak: The sad feeling you get when things don't go the way you want.

"Hitting the 'Wall:'" The point, during a walk or run, where your leg muscles have used up all available "quick-energy" molecules ("glycogen") and must turn to stored fat if you're going to keep moving.

Hold-back: Number of calories your body stops bringing out of storage for non-survival functions during periods of starvation (see also: **Cutback**).

Housekeeping Calories: Energy used to rebuild muscles and restock them with "fuel" following exercise; often overlooked when evaluating effectiveness of a particular exercise.

Infallible: What mommies and daddies are, until we become one.

Keister: Main contact point between couch potato and his vehicle of choice.

La-la Land: Where you go, to dream (see, for contrast: **Ca-ca County**).

Lap: Once around a walking "loop."

Laws of Eating: The more you eat, the more you
                    want to eat,
                    need to eat,
                    can eat.

The less you eat, the less you
            want to eat,
            need to eat,
            can eat.

Life-expectancy Chart: A reminder that there's more to being fit and losing bodysize than just **looking** good!

Lobotomy: A brain operation that increases one's appreciation of vegetables.

"Loop:" A "closed" (start/finish line the same) walking circuit (see also: **Lap**).

Loophole: Something you can slip through when nobody's looking.

Losing Bodysize: Something done, a) with great difficulty, by crushing your mind and body in a vise ("starvation diet"), or b) with great ease, by putting one foot in front of the other every day.

Losing Weight: What you do temporarily on a "diet."

Losing Size: What you do permanently when you walk yourself fit.

Lottery: Game of chance which millions play but, statistically speaking, no one ever wins (see also: **Starvation Diet**).

Magic: When something happens that defies rational explanation; in other words, something that **can't** happen (see also: **Miracle**).

Metabolic Furnaces: Exercised muscles, which give excess calories a chance to be burned rather than stored.

Millennium: One thousand years.

Miracle: Something that happens that defies rational explanation (see also: **Magic**).

Money's-worth: What you should get from things that **enrich** your life, not **destroy** it.

Moon: Big chunk of rock that stays within a few hundred thousand miles of Earth for some reason.

Mother Lode: Literally: richest vein of precious-metal ore; figuratively: where the best results are to be found (see also: **Fitwalking**).

Mother Teresa: A saintly woman (1910-97) who worked with the poor of India; winner of the 1979 Nobel Peace Prize.

"Murphy" Storehouses: Places where you would most like bodysize to leave, so it doesn't (see also: **Non-"Murphy" Storehouses**).

Murphy's Law (General): "If anything can go wrong, it will."

Murphy's Law of Bodysize Loss: Wherever you really want the bodysize to leave, that's where it won't.

Muscle: Protein-rich structure where the majority of calories that enter the body are burned (see also: **Metabolic Furnaces**).

National Debt: A number so high no one can count to it.

Niagara: Enormous waterfalls at the U. S.-Canadian border in upstate New York.

Non-"Murphy" Storehouses: Places where you don't care if they get thin, so they do so right away (see also: **"Murphy" Storehouses**).

Obsession: Stronger-than-normal dedication to doing something.

Objective Measurements: Things measured with respect to some "object" — stopwatch, yardstick, etc. (see also: **Subjective Impressions**).

Odds-on Choice: Overwhelming favorite to do something— usually: win a race..

On the Mark: Ready to exercise.

On the Shelf: Where exercisers who overdo it tend to wind up.

One-for-One Exchange: Where your body burns a calorie for every one your "diet" denies it (see also: **Two-for-One Exchange**).

One-in-a-Million: The number of people who will get struck by lightning in their lifetime and/or who will be harmed by trying to walk themselves fit.

Overkill: More happening than you expected to happen.

Oxygen Tent: Plastic enclosure for providing higher-than-normal amounts of oxygen to critically-ill people.

"Papayas-and-Pork Rinds:" Nonsensical "diet" that millions of plus-sized people will someday go on.

"Papayas-and-Prune Juice:" Alternate selection of the "'Diet' of the Month" Club.

Performance Charts: Records that people keep, to track the progress they're making.

Photographs: Objects that "freeze" time; useful for measuring otherwise undetectable changes.

Physical Fireworks: Bodily changes (stomach-churning; gut longing; etc.) that make you crave certain things.

Pipedream Pound: Amount of daily weight loss that "miracle diets" promise (see, for contrast: **Guaranteed Ounce**).

Power Molecules: Biochemicals that give you quick energy (see: **Glycogen**).

Primary Goals (of Fitwalking): Beautifying leg muscles and stengthening heart muscle (see also: **Side Effect [of Thinwalking]**).

Pro-survival: Anything that increases your chances of seeing tomorrow (see also: **Exercise**; see, for contrast: **Anti-survival**).

Protein: Major ingredient of muscle tissue.

Psychologists: People who try to figure out what's going on inside their own heads so they can tell you what's going on in yours.

Real-world Slimming: Something which happens in ounces-per-day of bodysize (see, for contrast: **Dream-world Slimming**).

Rolls: Bakery products that get better with butter.

"Rolls:" Aftermarket body parts that **don't** get better with butter.

Scrooge, Ebenezer: Main character in Charles Dickens's "A Christmas Carol;" known for overall meanness (see also: **Starvation Diet**).

Session: A relatively-prolonged time period, during which you do one thing almost exclusively.

"747:" Large aircraft that, ideally, goes higher and higher on take-off.

Seventh Tear: The point at which it becomes impossible to continue tearing paper.

Sherman, Gen. Wm. T.: Union General in the American Civil War (1861-65), who burned most of Georgia while conquering it.

Shortfall: The difference between what you need or want and what you actually get.

Side Effect: The unavoidable consequence of trying to achieve a primary effect.

Side effect (of Fitwalking): Bodysize loss.

Size-pound: The amount of size (space) a pound of body fat takes up.

Slave: Having your life under the control of someone or something else.

Sore: An "ache-y" feeling in muscles, tendons, etc., due to those things being torn down but not yet rebuilt.

Sports Watches: Clever little timepieces that give you more information than IBM mainframes used to.

Starvation: Death due to lack of food.

Starvation Diet: A time-honored way to take off 20 pounds and put back 30!

Starvation Patrol: Imaginary group of people empowered to arrest Mommies who don't feed their children every 20 or 30 seconds.

Step Test: Method for evaluating heart function.

Subconscious Mind: Portion of your brain designed to help you solve problems; receives strongest programming in infancy; therefore, "solutions" are often "infantile," and bear little relation to what would **really** solve the problem.

Survival Level (of Body Function): Calories used to keep heart beating, lungs breathing, kidneys filtering, etc. (see also: **Thrival Level**).

Tabloid: Newspaper, sold mainly in supermarkets, that tells us what we want to hear (see also: **Politician**.)

Targets: Performance goals.

"10 K:" Ten kilometers (= 6.21 miles.)

Thrival Level (of Body Function): Calories used for higher-level activities: problem-solving, rapid or prolonged movement, etc. (see, for contrast: **Survival Level**).

Time-lapse Camera: Device for detecting motion in apparently-immobile objects (plants, usually.)

Tortoise: Slow-moving animal of fable who always wins the race against the faster hare, presumably because of his concentration on the task at hand.

Two-for-One Exchange: What Fitwalking provides: every "unit" you walk gives you two "units" of benefit (see also: **One-for-one Exchange**).

Water: What your body surrounds salt molecules with, to keep them from killing you; therefore, the first thing your body eliminates when you remove salt from your diet, as you do on every "diet."

Zero: The number of times you should weigh yourself, in the course of a lifetime.

Zombie: The "living dead" (see also: **Starvation Diet**).

Appendix A

A New Term

When you go on a "diet," you lose weight, which is measured in "pounds."

When you **walk** yourself fit, on the other hand, you might **not** lose any weight; you might only lose **size**, which you **can't** measure in "pounds."

However, every pound of **weight** ("fat") takes up a certain amount of **space** (has a certain size), so if you lost that amount of **size,** it would be as if you'd lost that amount of **weight** (fat), no matter how much **actual** weight you'd lost.

For a variety of reasons, it would be nice to have some way to equate the amount of **size** you lose by Fitwalking with the amount of **weight** you would have lost if you'd dieted yourself down to that same size. In fact, there is such a way, through a term we call a **"size-pound,"** which is nothing more than

the amount of space that a pound of fat takes up.

Since, with Fitwalking, all we care about is losing "space" ("size"), all we're interested in is "size-pounds:" how many you've lost; how many you'd still like to lose; etc.

When you go on a "diet," you say: "I'd like to lose 40 pounds."

With Fitwalking, you say: "I'd like to lose 40 size-pounds," which is the amount of size you would lose if you lost 40 pounds of fat, regardless how much weight you'll **actually** be losing."

To use myself as an example:

If I "diet" myself down to 160 pounds, from a starting weight of 200, I can fit into Size 32 slacks; I would have lost 40 size-pounds, which, as it happens, is the same number of **actual** pounds I lost, since I did it all through dieting.

However, if I **walk** myself down from the same starting point, I can get into those Size 32 slacks at a scale weight of **175**, because I didn't just **lose** the fat, I "converted" a lot of it into muscle, which is **not weightless**.

In the second case, even though I've lost only 25 **actual** pounds, I would still have lost the same 40 "size-pounds." In other words, I will have gotten down to the same **size** as I would have if I had simply lost 40 **pounds**!

Since body size is all I care about, "size-pounds" are the only things that matter.

In other words: I wouldn't care if I **gained** 50 actual pounds by walking; as long as I lost 40 **size**-pounds and could fit into those Size 32 slacks, the program would have done its job!

So don't worry about actual pounds. Just worry about losing bodysize—measured, if necessary, in "size-pounds—" and you'll be "home free!"

Appendix B

Pedometer Walking

So you've started walking yourself fit.

At which point, you ask the question virtually **every** new walker asks:

"Gee: I wonder if there's any way to tell how **far** I'm walking every day—at work, at home, at school, wherever —without packing a tape measure the size of a **firehose** on my back?!"

The answer?

Yes, there is—and it doesn't involve tape measures or firehoses or anything you need the neighborhood burro to haul around!

All it takes is a little device known as a "pedometer," which you clip to your belt or waistband—or stick in your pocket or purse, if you have one of the newer **tri-axis** models—and just start walking.

What happens then is, the pedometer starts recording how many steps you're taking, and, if you've bought one of the spiffier models: the distance you're walking, the number of calories you're burning, etc.

And what happens then?

Well, can we speak confidentially: you get "hooked" on the little guy: you can't wait to pop it open every night—or press the "magic button"—and see how far you've walked that day.

Is that bad: to be addicted to something like a pedometer?

I don't know: depends on how long you plan on living, since "walkers" tend to live a whole lot longer than non-walkers, so the more a pedometer says you've walked each day, the longer you're likely to live, all else being equal.

So, if that's "bad," would someone please show me the way to "**awful**?!"

Obviously, there's **nothing** wrong with being "addicted" to pedometer walking, any more than there is with being "addicted" to fresh air!

So, the only question is: Which pedometer to buy?

Well, hopefully, we've taken the guesswork out of that for you:

Having tested virtually every pedometer known to man, we finally found one that combines everything we were looking for in a pedometer: quality, readability, ease of programming, accuracy, appearance, etc. And that one is the model HJ-320, from Omron Healthcare, which measures steps, distance, calories burned, features a digital clock and, most important, a 7-day memory, so that, with the flick of a button, you can compare today's results with yesterday's, two days ago, three days ago, etc.

Of course, whichever pedometer you choose, we know you'll be walking—and pedometering—for a lifetime, and know you'll come to get as much of a kick out of your pedometer as you do out of your daily Fitwalk.

For now, though, you'll have to excuse me while I—that's right: push the "magic button," to see how far I've walked today.

Which is: Wow—that far?!

Fantastic!

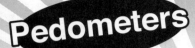
Audio Books

Pedometers

CD Programs
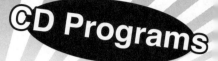

SUPER WEB SPECIALS!

Volume Discounts

Children's Books

eBooks

Posters

ORDERING INFORMATION

1) Log on to **MoonRiverPublishing.com**
2) Click the **"Store"** tab on the Home page
3) Click the **"Add to Cart"** tab under the product(s) you want
4) Enter **WYF45786** in the "Coupon Code" box
5) Click **"Apply"**; **$5 discount** will automatically be applied to each item ordered
6) Click **"Checkout"**
7) Enter personal information (name, address, etc.) and payment information on **Checkout** page, then click **"Submit"**

- eBook and Audio Book files will be emailed to you.
- CD programs, pedometers, etc., will be sent by regular mail.